Kind Karma® Kids Yoga

Awaken Your Inner Shaman

With Yoga, Meditation, Breathing Exercises & Visualization

√ Tap into Animal Prana Power
√ Align with Nature's Wisdom & Healing Energy

All graphic designs, illustrations, diagrams and charts in this book were created by Dean Telano

By **Dean Telano**, Ph.D., E-RYT 500, RCYT, RPYT
Author of "Kind Karma Worldwide™: Inspirational Quotes & Empowering Thoughts for Raising the Vibration of Humanity"

KIND KARMA® KIDS YOGA

AWAKEN YOUR INNER SHAMAN

WITH YOGA, MEDITATION, BREATHING EXERCISES AND VISUALIZATION

TAP INTO YOUR ANIMAL PRANA
ALIGN WITH NATURE'S WISDOM AND HEALING ENERGY

Author: Dean Telano, Ph.D., E-RYT 500, RCYT, RPYT, YACEP, KKRGM-24
Founder of Kind Karma Worldwide™
Creator of Kind Karma® Yoga, Rahini Yoga®, Kind Karma® Kids Yoga,
Awaken Qigong & Awaken with Meditation

All graphic designs, illustrations, diagrams and charts in this book were created by Dean Telano

Edited by: Naomi Miller-Telano & Heidi Zeller

Published by: Kind Karma Publications

Kind Karma® Yoga
www.kindkarmayoga.com

Copyright 2022. All rights reserved. No part of this book may be reproduced, including graphic illustrations and designs, by any means without written permission of the author.

ISBN: 978-0-9846625-1-7

Printed in the United States of America

"Kind Karma® Yoga doesn't begin on the mat; it begins in your heart."

– Dr. Dean Telano, Creator of Kind Karma® Yoga & Kind Karma® Kids Yoga

Contents

Introduction..7

Section I

Kind Karma Kids Yoga Nature Poses
"Align with Nature's Wisdom & Healing Energy"
Yoga Poses to Develop a Kinship with Nature

Blossoming Lotus Pose..14
Five Pointed Star Pose...16
Half Moon Rising Pose...18
Mountain Pose...20
Rainbow Breathing Pose...22
Rainbow Pose...24
Sun Salute...26
Tree Hug Pose..28
Volcano Pose & Lava Flows..30
Waterfall Pose..32

Section II

Kind Karma Kids Yoga Animal Poses
"Tap into the Animal Prana Power"

Bear Pose..36
Blissful Otter Pose...40
Buffalo Pose..42
Butterfly Pose...46
Cat Pose..50
Caterpillar Pose..54
Cobra Pose..58

Cow Pose..62
Crocodile Pose...66
Crow Pose..70
Deer Pose...74
Dog Pose..78
Eagle Pose..82
Fish Pose..86
Flamingo Pose...90
Frog Pose...94
Hedgehog Pose..98
Horse Pose...102
Jellyfish Pose 106
Kangaroo Pose..110
Lion's Breath Pose..114
Lizard Pose..118
Locust Pose...122
Monkey Leaping Pose..126
Mouse Pose...130
Pigeon Pose...134
Tiger Pose..138
Turtle Pose..142
Whale Pose..146
Wolf Pose...150
Yoga Pose / Associated Animal Attributes..........154

Section III

Kind Karma Kids Yoga Salutations, Root With Salutes and Flows

Sun Salutations..160
Tree Salutations...166
4- Element Warrior Flow....................................168

I-Am-My-Breath Affirmation Warrior Flow..169
The Power of My Inner Shaman..170
Warrior Poses..171

Section IV

Kind Karma Kids Breathing Exercises (Pranayama) And Meditation Techniques

Prana Power..176
Animal & Nature Breathing Exercises..177
Dog Panting Breath..179
Rainbow Breath Moving Meditation..180
4-Word Finger Meditation..181
Heart Breath Meditation..182
White Light Meditation: 7 Sacred Directions..183

Section V

Kind Karma Kids Yoga: Medicine Wheels, Seven Sacred Directions, Four Elements, Crystals

Medicine Wheels..186
The Four Elements of Nature's Magic..190
The Four Elements of the Human Body..192
Crystals & the 4 Elements..194
The Seven Sacred Directions of the Medicine Wheel..195
Key Aspects of the Medicine Wheel for Lesson Plans..196

References..197
About the Author..198

Introduction

Kind Karma Kids Yoga Inner Shaman Practice

This book was created so anyone with or without yoga experience can learn how to develop a kinship with yoga, animals, and nature. You will soon discover this book is easy to follow, fun to learn, amazingly contemporary, and what we feel is needed for the world. Included are visual and breathtaking graphic designs that embody "nature" yoga poses and "animal" yoga poses designed to embrace the energy (Sanskrit: prana) of Mother Earth and her inhabitants. Furthermore, this book contains vibrant illustrations and directions for yoga salutations, root with salutes, flows, meditation, breathwork, when to use crystals, and how to use the American Native Medicine Wheel, Four Elements and Seven Sacred Directions with yoga. You will find invaluable resources to guide children of ages 3 to 16 to find confidence, inner strength, determination, and coping skills needed to navigate through daily challenges in life.

As a comprehensive Kind Karma Kids Yoga Inner Shaman Practice, *this book offers step-by-step directions of uniquely designed graphic images, charts, illustrations and tables, and* life-changing affirmations *that pertain to specific positive animal attributes and charts of healing crystals that match the vibrational energies of nature and, what we call –* animal prana power.

Moreover, this book is truly a resource for everyone: from the parent with little or no yoga knowledge to the private or group therapist or school teacher who wants to learn breath meditation, introduce color therapy and to help children with self-regulation management. For the yoga teacher, you will have at your fingertips moment themes ideas, and class concepts or lesson plans to use.

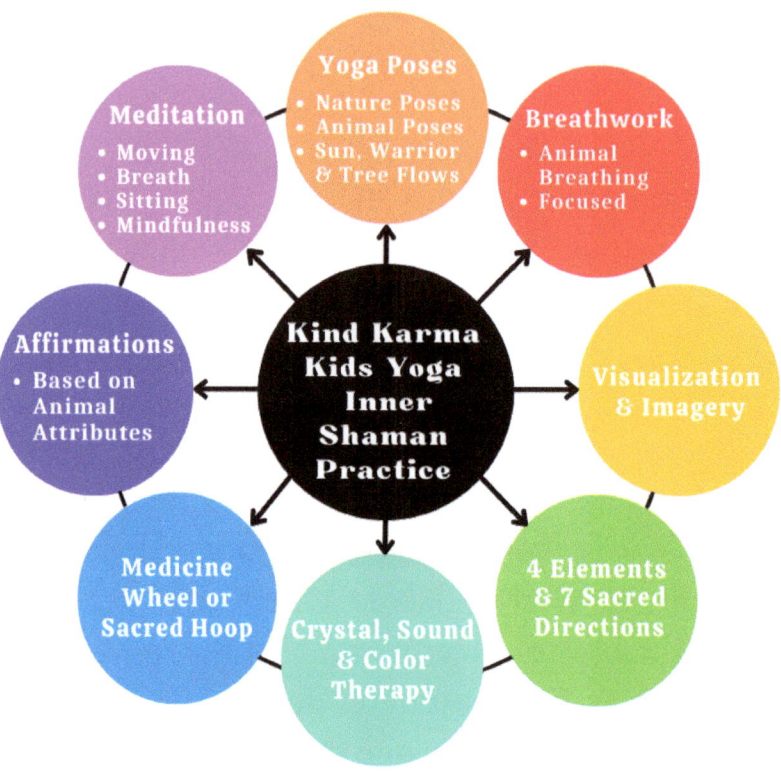

A Depiction of the Eight Healing Modalities of the Kind Karma Kids Yoga Inner Shaman Practice

As shown in the above wheel chart, to devise a *Kind Karma Kids Yoga Shaman Practice,* the author Dr. Dean Telano uses Yoga Poses, Breathwork, Meditation, Visualization & Imagery, the 4 Elements and 7 Sacred Directions, Crystal & Sound Healing, Medicine Wheel, and Affirmations. All the nature and animal poses have detailed descriptions of how to practice the poses, listed benefits of the poses, affirmations, fun facts and crystal usage to contribute to a child's connection to nature. The *Inner Shaman Practice* reminds us that nature often acts like a mirror that reflects who and what we are, how we are impacting the planet, and more importantly, what we are becoming as individuals. This practice emphasizes the human and nature relationship and its worldwide impact.

HOW TO USE THE BOOK

First and foremost this book is all about having fun, so have lots of it when you are reading, sharing or following this book! Afterall, it's a *kids yoga* book.

Now, let's get into developing your *Kind Karma Kids Yoga Inner Shaman Practice!* Below, you will find suggestions on how to navigate all this book has to offer.

Step #1

The best way to begin is to thoroughly review the 10 "nature" poses and the 30 "animal" poses found in Sections I & II. See if you can connect with the energy of each image. Can you energetically *feel* the landscape, breadth and the width of each image? Perhaps you can get a sense of the *prana* intertwined in each image. After going through an image, can you see how the affirmations are related to each nature or animal pose? If not, we recommend you review the "associated animal attributes" tables. This will be a great help.

Step #2

As already mentioned, after you become acquainted with the yoga poses in Sections I & II, read and review the chart on the *"associated animal attributes."* For example, if you were to go to the animal attribute table and locate "dog", you will see one of the attributes for a dog is "loving" (please notice that "loving" is also part of the affirmation on the *dog pose* image). This will help you to create your yoga practice by choosing and matching the poses and the specific attributes you would like the child, student or client to embody.

Step #3

At this point, it is advisable to look at the crystal chart in Section V. This chart shows how to use crystals for personal use, for yoga practice, class lesson plans and to deepen the connection with Mother Earth.

Step #4

Determine which meditation technique you would like to incorporate into your lesson found in Section IV. In this section, you will find breathing exercises (*"pranayama"*) and various meditation practices. Sticking with our prior dog theme, you will find *"Dog Panting Breath"*. This is so much fun, and kids love to imitate how a dog breathes. For the mom, counselor or teacher, *"The Rainbow Breath Moving Meditation"*, uses visualization, imagery and color therapy to reduce stress and anxiety, and to channel pent-up energy. To offer another example, *"Animal & Nature Breathing Exercises" to promote Nature Interconnectedness & Self-Regulation"*: in Section IV, details instructions of how to use specific breathing techniques that correspond to specific animals. These lists are a foundational resource, especially for the younger age children who love to explore connections with animals.

Step #5

Medicine Wheel

Read and learn about the *Medicine Wheel*. If this information is new to you, take your time, invite the moment to absorb and learn the material, and discover new ways to be creative. There are five medicine wheels in the book and all are presented with explanations and teaching ideas.

The Medicine Wheel charts are circular in nature. The significance of the Circle Shape and its relationship to the Medicine Wheel is often used in Kind Karma Yoga. We call the "circle shape" – "The Circle of Light & Compassion" and that's why we often put kids in a circle, as they are learning about yoga in the context of the Medicine Wheel, or as the Native Amercians call it, the *Sacred Hoop*. This information will serve you well for your yoga class themes. Another useful fact is that the Medicine Wheel represents the "sun", which can be used with your "sun" themed classes or lessons. Still discussing the Medicine Wheel, Medicine Wheel #4 *"Animal Breathing"*, offers breathing techniques associated with individual animals. These breathing techniques are fun and exciting, adding to a successful outcome of your practice goals. Another such example can be found on Medicine Wheel #5, which offers creative themes incorporating the animal pose, attributes, and crystals.

Four Elements of Nature's Magic

You will find an illustrated diagram of *"The Four Elements of Nature's Magic"*, and *"The Four Elements of the Human Body"*. Here are explanations of the four elements, and where they are found in the body. Here, you will learn that connecting with the earth, water, fire, and air elements within us, will help the yoga student to deepen their connection with nature.

Seven Sacred Directions

This is an integral part of the *Inner Shaman Practice* because we are teaching the student that there are more than 4 directions. In the Native American culture, or from a shamanistic point of view, there exists Seven Sacred Directions. We teach this important concept through visualization, color therapy and meditation, and this is found in the *White Light Meditation: 7 Sacred Directions* illustration. Furthermore, it's also mentioned in the illustration, *"Seven Sacred Directions of the Medicine Wheel or Sacred Hoop.*

Step #6

Finally, the last step is to have fun, play, teach, and to explore your own *Inner Shaman Practice*. Enjoy this journey through a shamanistic and holistic approach to healing with yoga, meditation, crystals, and of course, *NATURE!*

SECTION I

Kind Karma Kids Yoga Nature Poses
"Align With Nature's Wisdom & Healing Energy"

Yoga Poses To Develop a Kinship With Nature

1. Blossoming Lotus Pose
2. Five Pointed Star Pose
3. Half Moon Rising Pose
4. Mountain Pose
5. Rainbow Breathing Pose
6. Rainbow Pose
7. Sun Salute
8. Tree Hug Pose
9. Volcano Pose & Lava Flows
10. Waterfall Pose

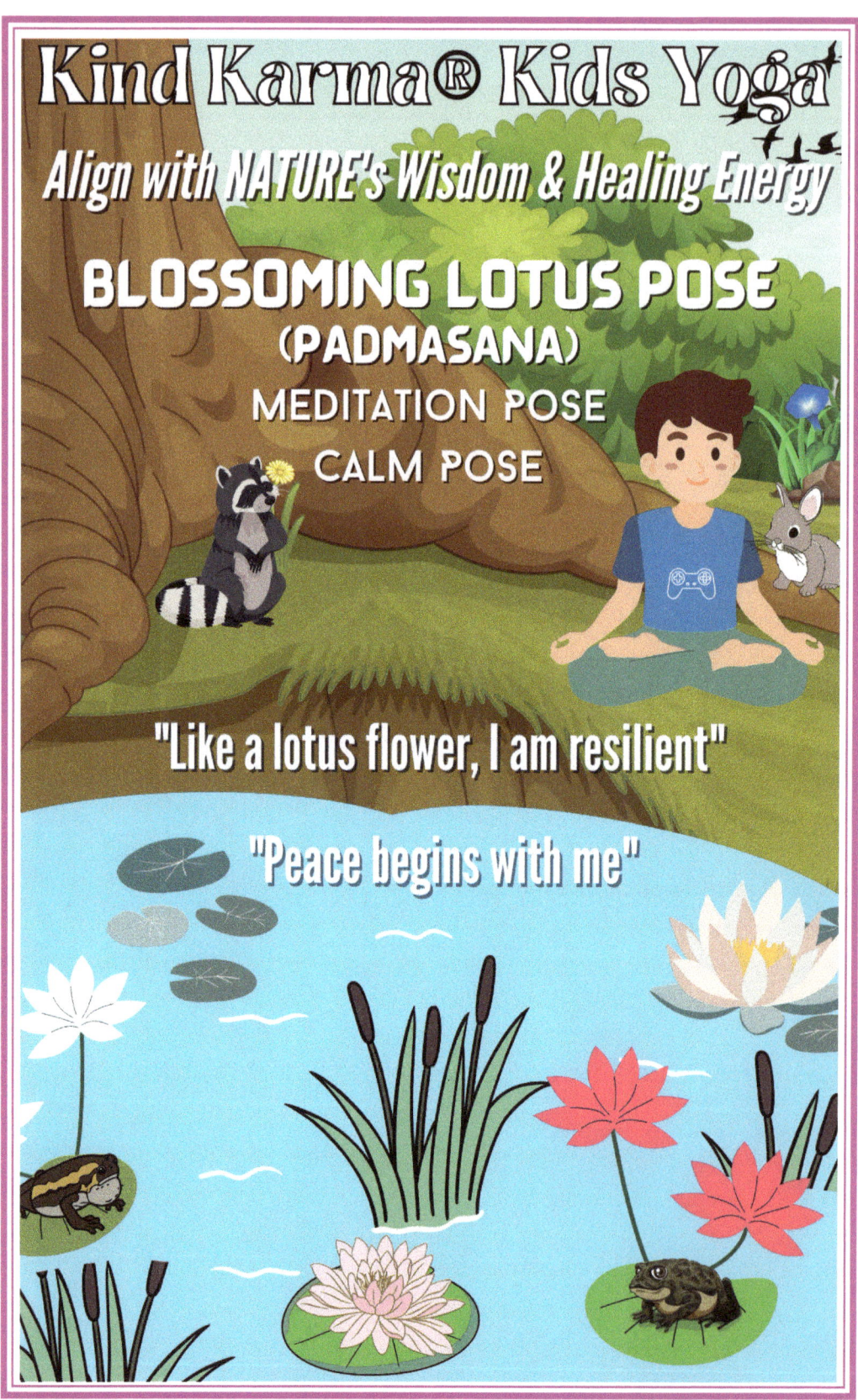

Blossoming Lotus Pose

1. Sit comfortably with your legs stretched out in front of the body.
2. Carefully bend one leg at a time and place your foot on top of the opposite thigh with the bottoms of each foot facing up. Each knee should be able to touch the ground.
   - If this is uncomfortable, practice Half-Lotus, where only one foot is on top of the thigh. Be sure to switch sides.
3. Place your hands on top of your knees palms up, gently touching the tips of your thumbs with the tips of your index fingers.
4. Close your eyes, and breathe slowly in this meditation pose.
5. Become a blossoming lotus flower by lengthening your spine real tall and reaching through the water to bloom in the sun.

Benefits

- Promotes calm and relaxation.
- Very grounding.
- Increases awareness.
- Keeps the spine straight and helps to develop good posture.
- Increasing flexibility in the hips and legs.

Fun Facts for Connecting Children with Nature

- The lotus seed can survive droughts for 200 years, then blossom.
- It's India's national flower (yoga originated in ancient India).

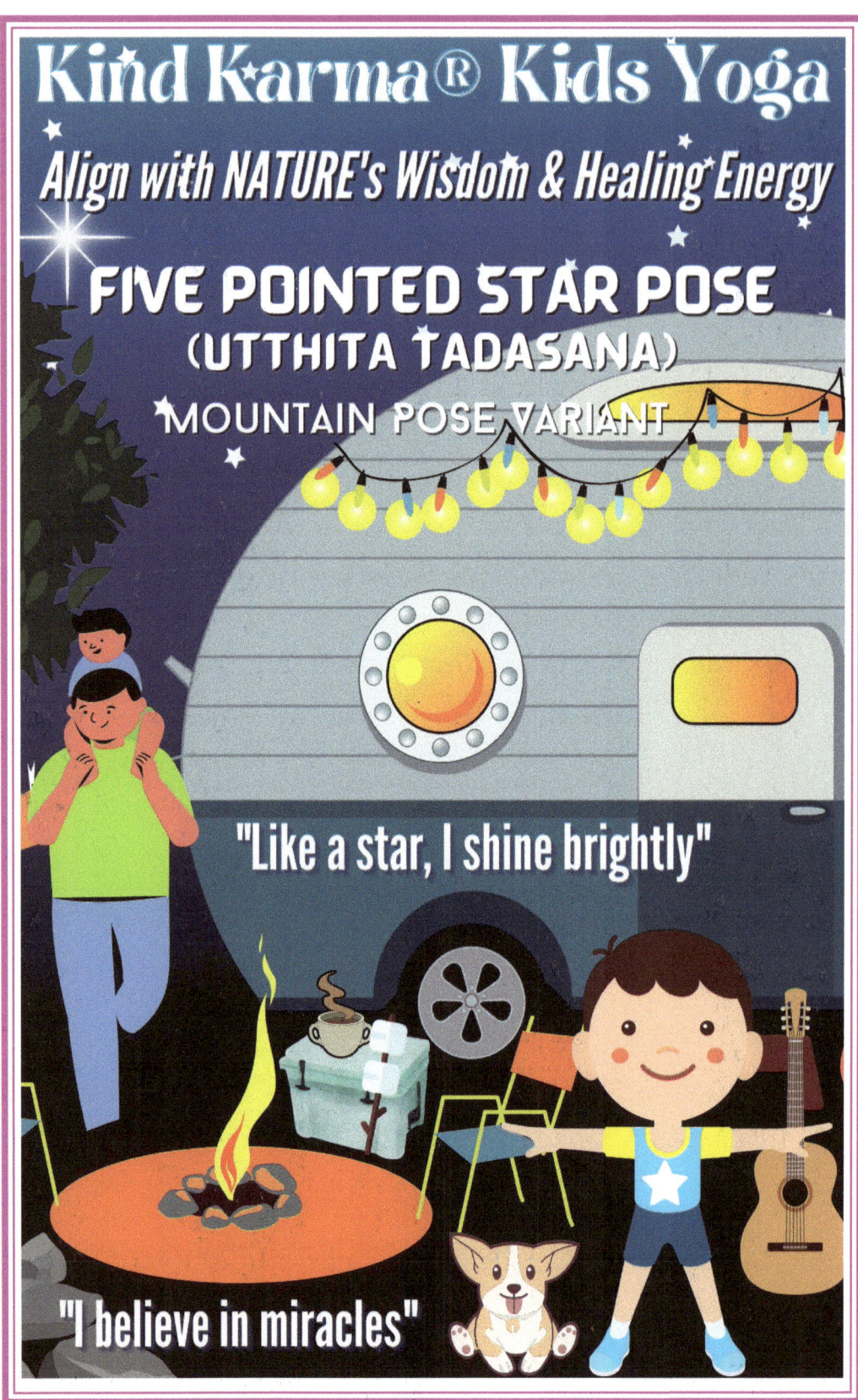

Five Pointed Star Pose

1. Begin in Mountain Pose.

2. Step your feet hip-width apart and stretch your arms out to your sides, shoulder height. Your body should be in a **star shape.**

    - Stay tall and keep the shoulders relaxed.
    - Expand your energy out through your fingers and toes.

3. Hold this pose for three to five deep breaths, then lower your arms back down and step your feet back together, in Mountain Pose.

Benefits

- Lengthens, opens and energizes the entire body.
- Works on core strength and balance.
- Stretches and opens the chest, improving posture and breathing.
- Increases concentration.
- Builds confidence.
- Encourages children to practice stillness in their own space.

Fun Facts for Connecting Children with Nature

- Every star you see in the night sky is bigger and brighter than our sun.
- It takes millions of years for a star's light to reach our eyes.

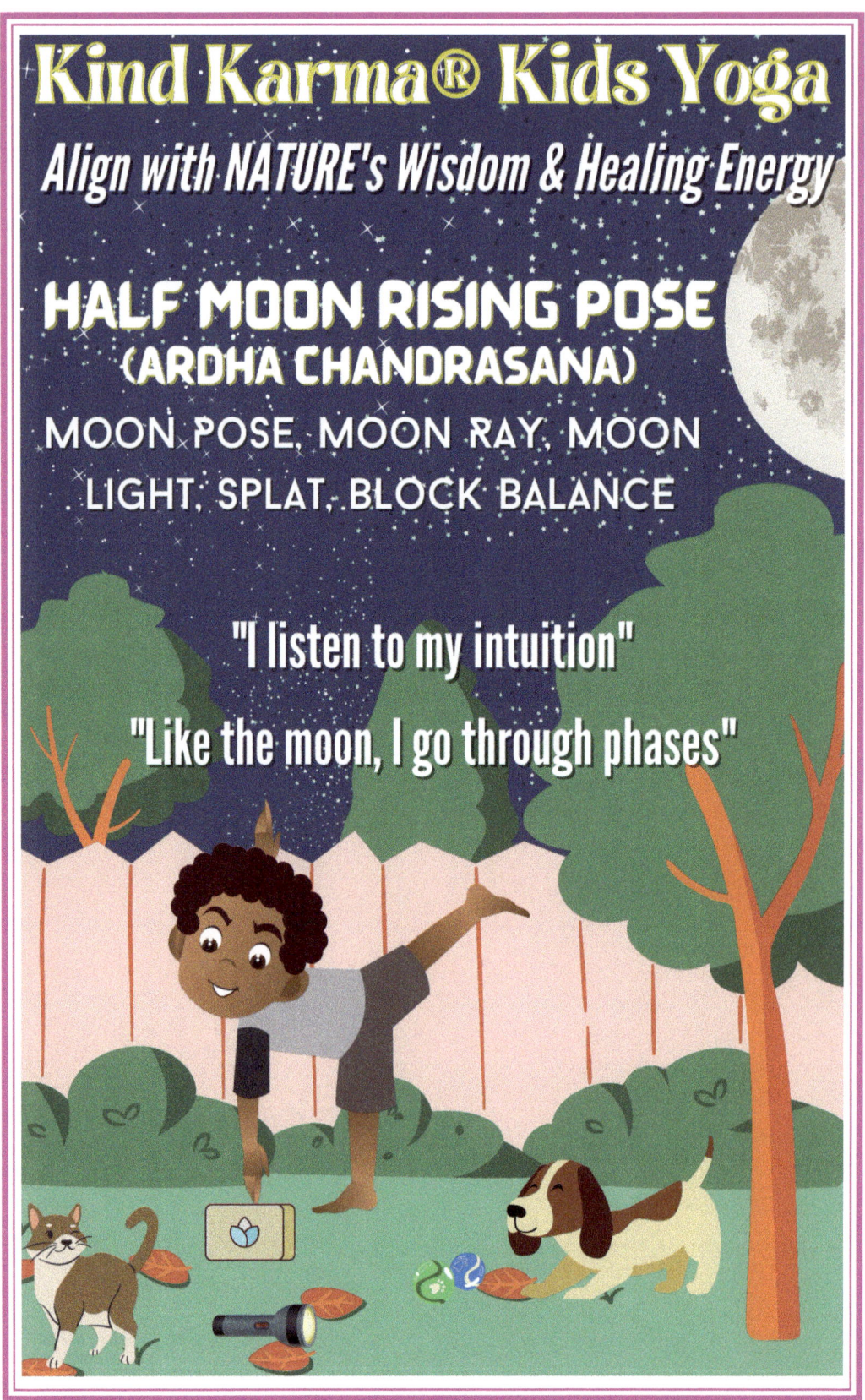

Half Moon Rising Pose

Using the Wall & Yoga Block Will Help You to Rise

1. Stand beside a wall with the right side of your body against it.

2. Slowly, place a yoga block down, right below your shoulder. As you lower the block, lift the left leg up and back towards the wall.

3. Try your best to keep your shoulders and back against the wall. Make sure the right foot is facing forward, as your body mirrors the image of the **half-moon rising.**

4. Hold for three to five breaths, then switch sides.

Benefits

- Improves balance and coordination, and increases proprioceptive awareness.
- Lengthens the spine, and opens the torso, chest and shoulders.
- Strengthens the core, legs, knees and ankles.
- Increases focus.
- Calms, cools, relieves stress and reduces anxiety.

Fun Facts for Connecting Children with Nature

- It takes the Moon about 27 days to orbit the planet Earth.
- The Moon is one of the main causes of tides on Earth.

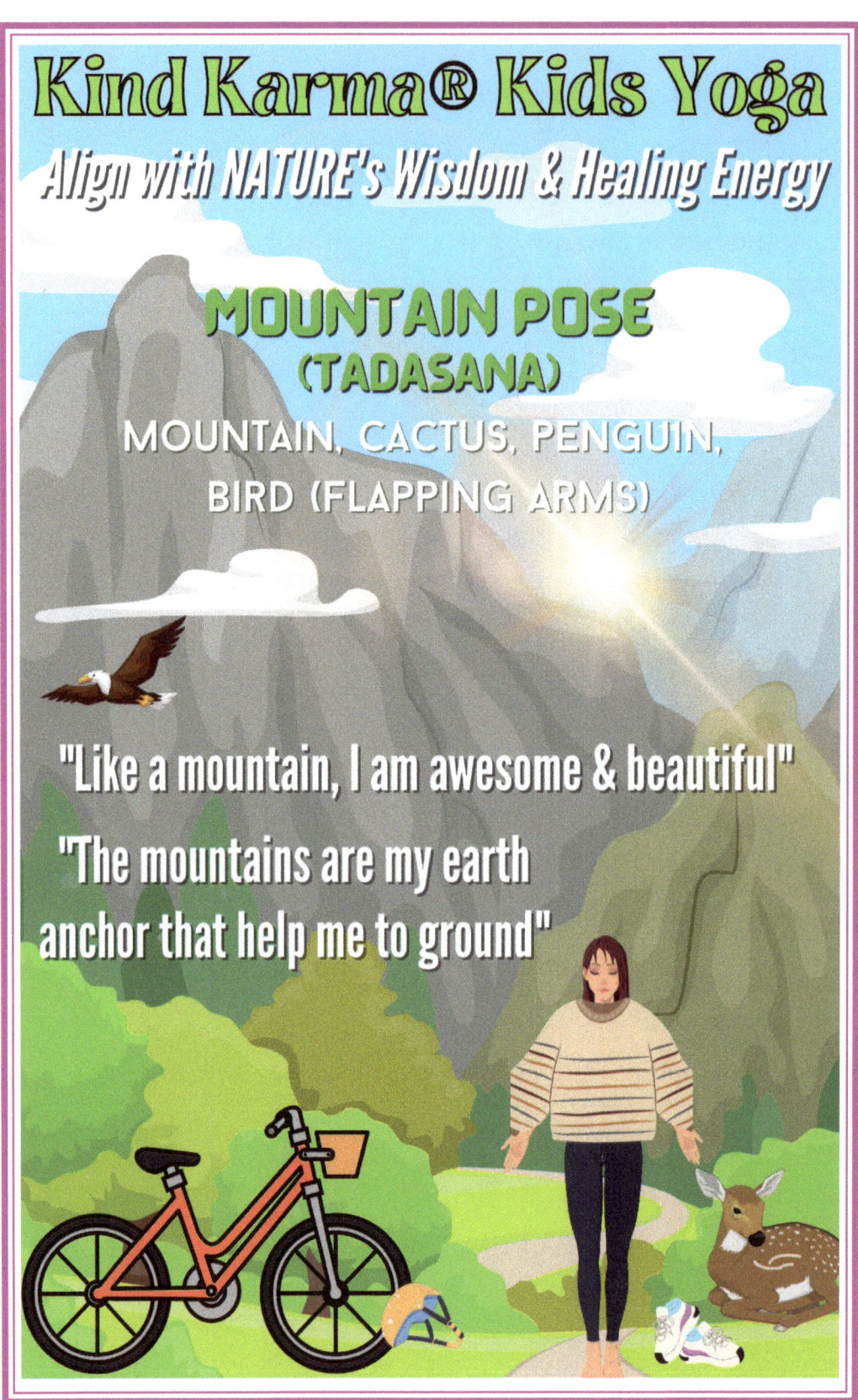

Mountain Pose

1. Stand tall, with your toes touching and heels slightly apart. Imagine you can grow the bottoms of your feet down into the Earth, which helps you feel strong and solid as a **mountain.**

    - Tip: To improve your balance, stand with your feet hip-width apart.

2. Feeling tall, gently press your shoulders back and allow your arms to fall by your sides.

3. Now, turn your palms forward, keeping your fingers lengthened.

4. Lengthen your spine by lifting the crown of your head toward the sky right above you.

5. Breathe deeply, holding the pose for three to five breaths.

Benefits

- Promotes calm and relaxation.
- Helps with grounding and centering.
- Promotes posture awareness.
- Improves balance and strengthens the core and legs.
- Encourages stillness and silence.

Fun Facts for Connecting Children with Nature

- Mount Everest is growing by about 6cm each year.
- Some of the highest mountains are at the bottom of the sea.

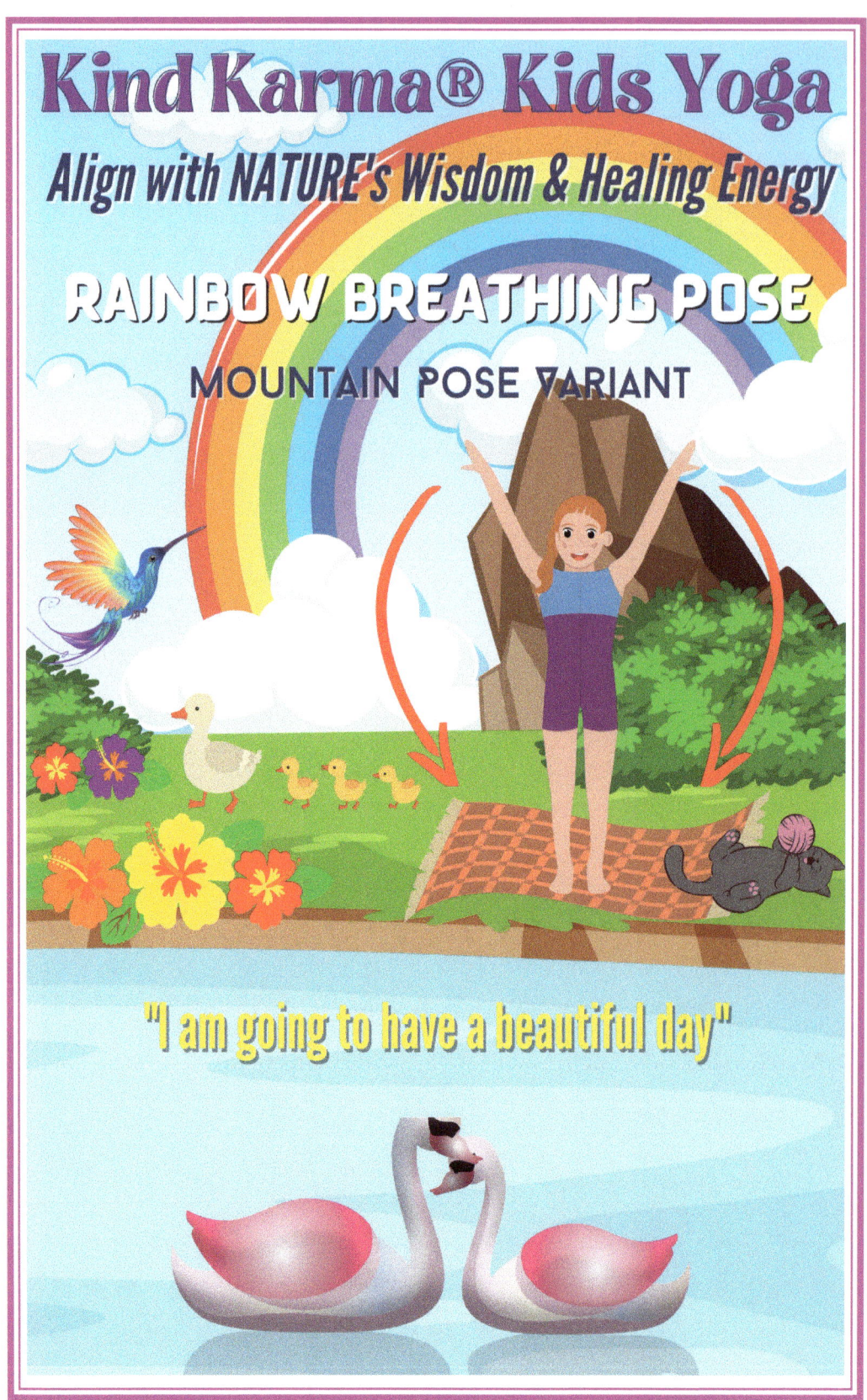

Rainbow Breathing Pose

1. Stand with your feet hip-width apart and arms down by the sides of your body.

2. From the sides of your body, swing your arms up to the sky. Imagine your arms/hands are creating a **rainbow** all around you.

   - You can visualize any color of the rainbow or have the children mix and match to create their own **rainbow.**

3. Inhale when you lift your arms, and exhale when you lower your arms. Breathe deeply.

4. Repeat as long as desired.

Benefits

- Redirects and channels excess energy or pent up emotional energy.
- Is a form of movement-based meditation.
- Promotes deep breathing and strengthens respiration.
- A form of self-regulation to manage stress or tension.
- A form of guided imagery or visualization.
- Increases awareness.

Fun Facts for Connecting Children with Nature

- You can't reach the end of the rainbow because a rainbow is sort of like an optical illusion.
- Earth is the only planet in our solar system with rainbows.

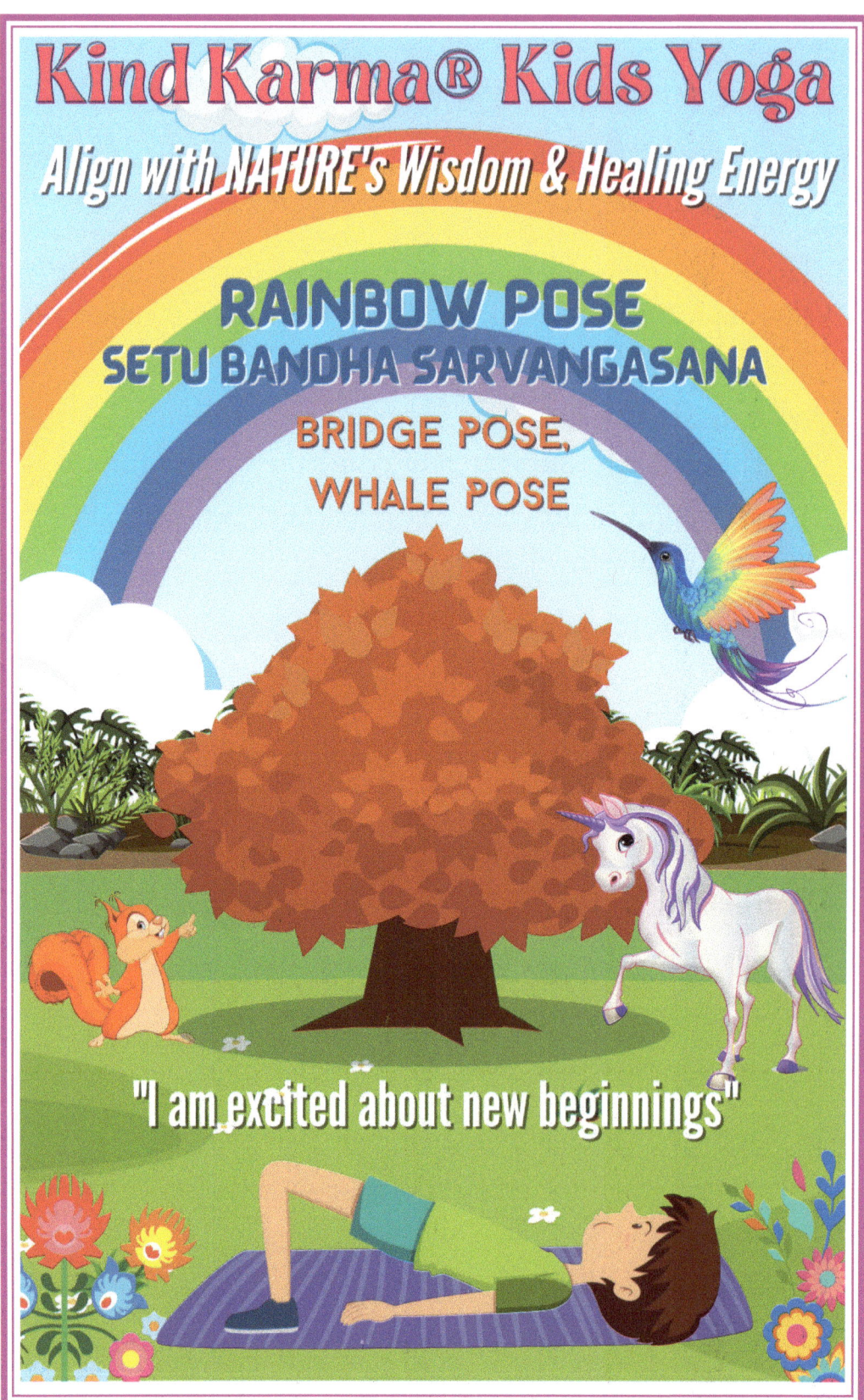

Rainbow Pose

1. Lay down on your back and place your arms on the floor alongside your body, with the palms facing down.

2. Bend your knees, and set your feet flat on the floor with your toes pointing straight ahead. Your knees should be hip-width apart.

3. Inhale and lift your hips towards the ceiling. Try to gently arch the spine (bridge) into a colorful **rainbow crescent shape**.

4. Hold for three to five breaths.

5. Exhale and slowly lower your hips back to the floor.

Benefits

- Helps to awaken the body.
- Increases spine flexibility and opens the chest, shoulders and hips.
- Strengthens the back and leg muscles.
- Clears and calms the mind.
- Reduces stress, anxiety and depression.

Fun Facts for Connecting Children with Nature

- On the ground, we can only see a semi-circle rainbow; however, if you look at it from an airplane, you can see a rainbow in a complete circle.
- Two people never see the same rainbow.

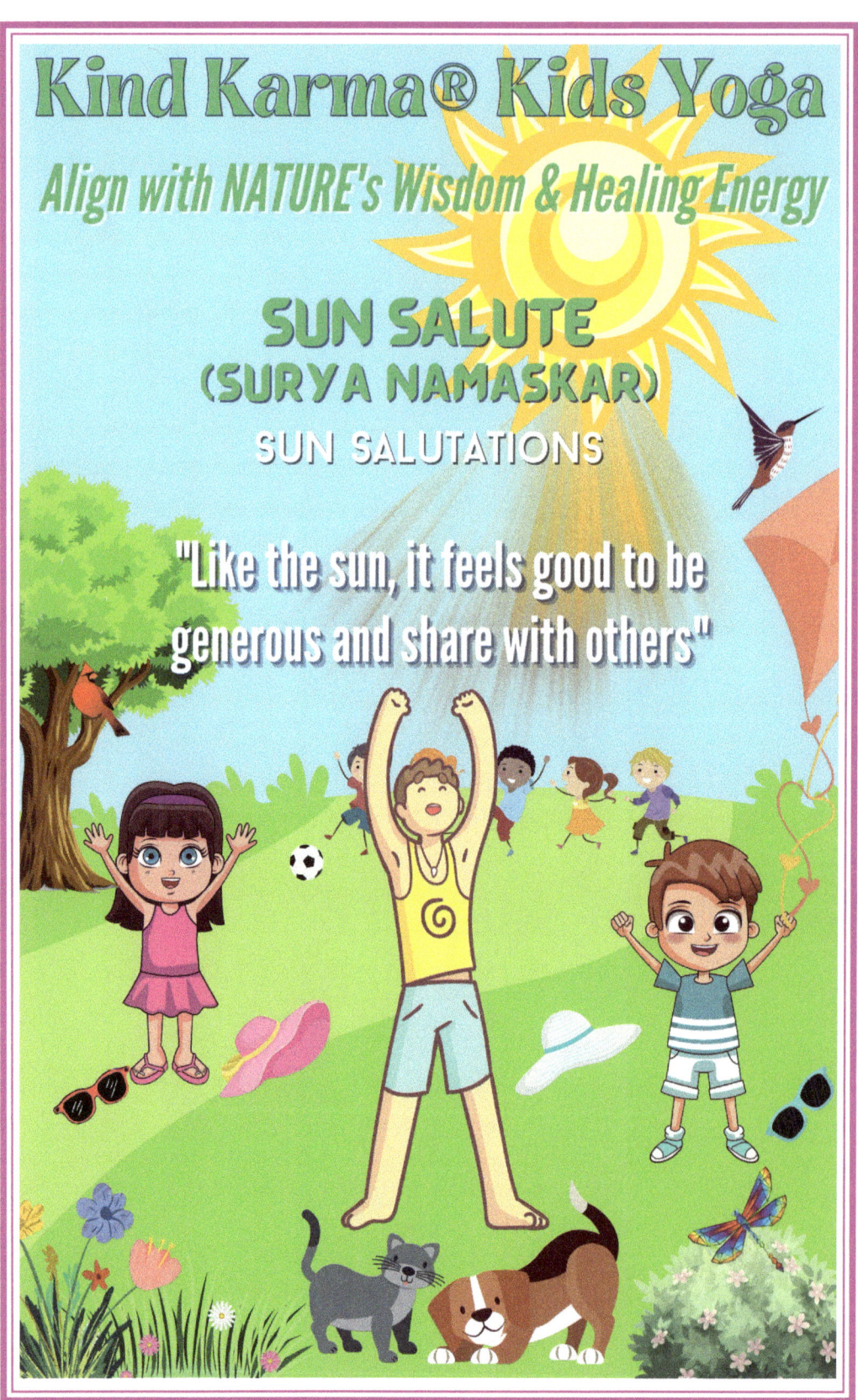

Sun Salute

- Refer to Sun Salutation Illustrations in Section III.

Benefits

- Awakens and energizes the body and increases endurance.
- Redirects and channels excess energy or pent up emotional energy.
- Increases flexibility and strength.
- Calms and clears the mind.
- Improves concentration and focus.
- Enhances memory power.
- A great way to teach how to link the breath to movement.

Fun Facts for Connecting Children with Nature

- The Sun is over 4.5 billion years old.
- The Sun's light reaches the Earth in about eight minutes.

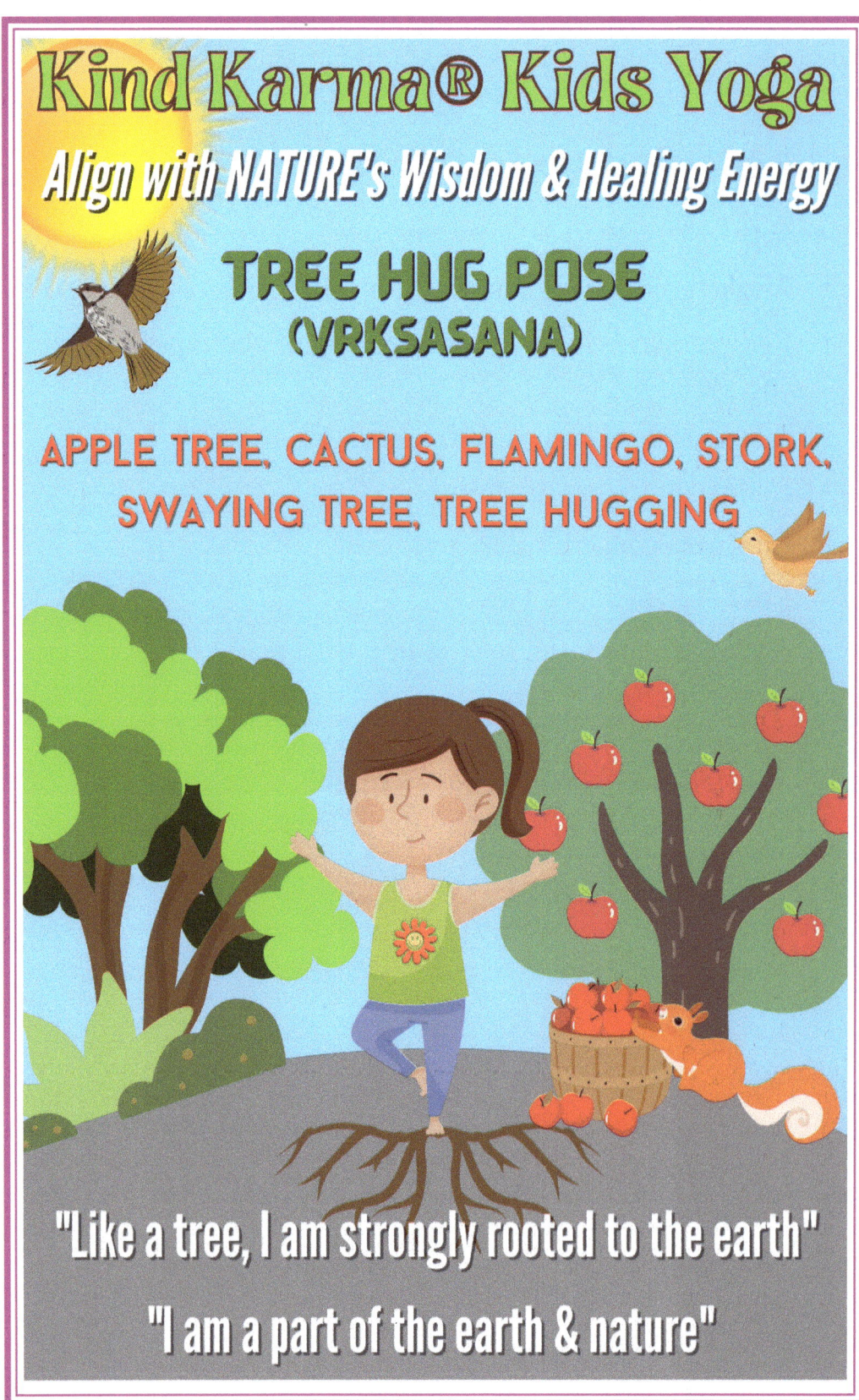

Tree Hug Pose

(Refer to the Tree Salutation Illustrations for Variations)

1. Begin in Mountain Pose. Look ahead and find a point to focus on.
2. Standing on your left leg, slowly bring up your right foot. Bend your knee, and place your right foot on the inside part of your left leg (avoid pressing your foot against the inside of your knee).
   - Modification: You can set your toes on the floor and your heel against your ankle.
3. As you ground and root your left leg and foot, lift and reach out your arms as if you were *hugging* a very wide **tree.**
4. Lengthening through your core, hold this pose for three to five breaths, then lower your arms down and stand on both legs.
5. Repeat on your opposite side.

Benefits

- Helps to develop balance skills and increase body awareness.
- Strengthens the core muscles and stabilizers.
- Increases strength on the standing leg.
- Improves concentration and focus.
- Calms the mind and nervous system.

Fun Facts for Connecting Children with Nature

- Trees are able to communicate with each other.
- Trees provide oxygen to help us breathe.

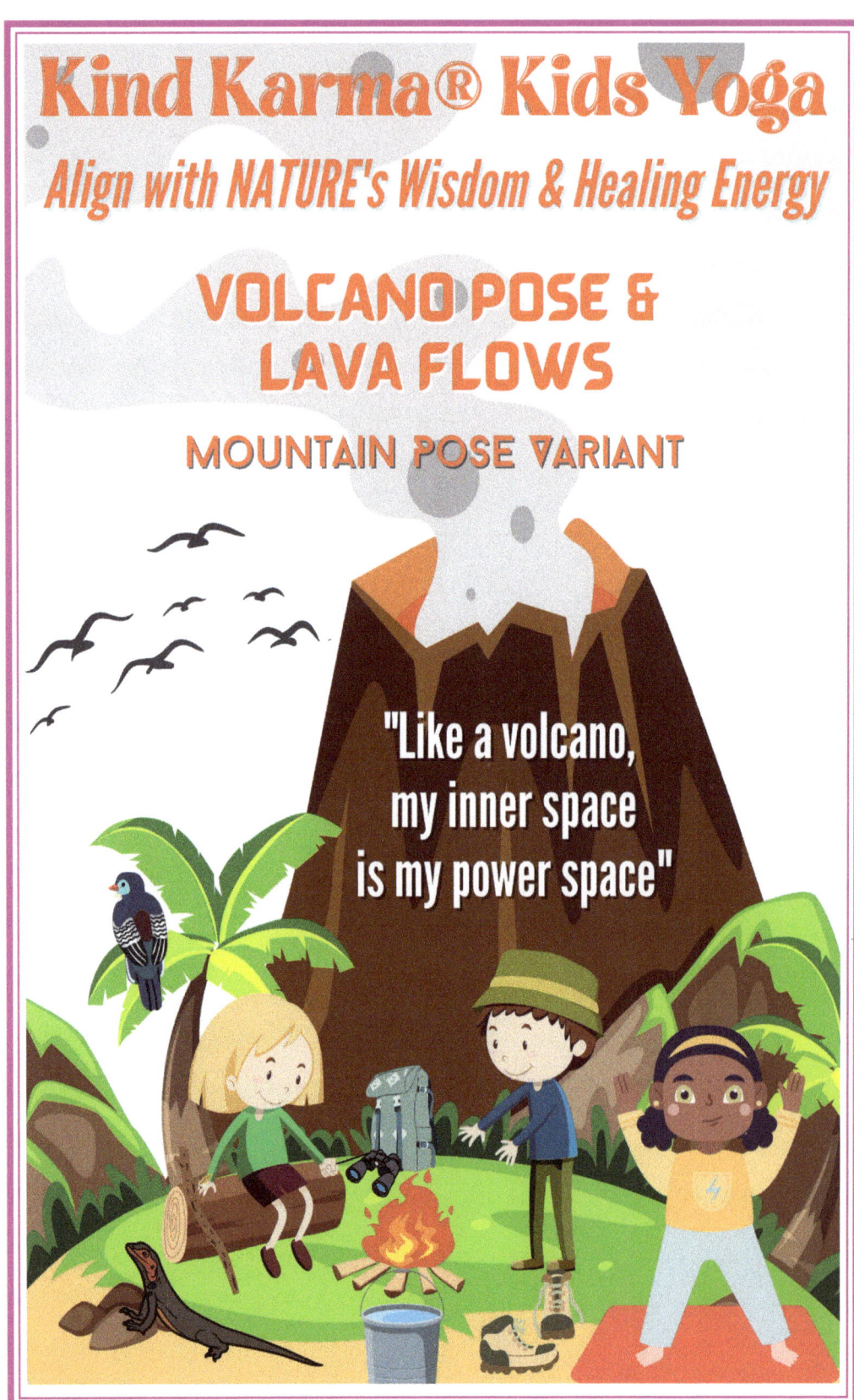

Volcano Pose & Lava Flows

1. Stand tall and strong in Mountain Pose.
2. Bend forward, reach down towards your toes and *find your lava*.
3. Roll slowly up, one vertebra at a time, imagining you are **lava** coming up through the **volcano.**
   - You can make **lava** sounds as you come up.
4. Erupt and release the **lava** by:

   (a) Shouting and jumping up into Five Pointed Star Pose, with your feet apart and reaching your arms wide and high.

   (b) Jumping your feet back together and arms back to your sides into Mountain Pose.
5. Repeat using your imagination by changing the pace and intensity.

Benefits

- Stretches the entire body and lengthens the spine.
- Strengthens the core, legs, back, shoulders and arms.
- Develops balance and coordination.
- Develops creativity, visualization and imagination.
- Redirects and channels excess energy or pent up emotional energy.

Fun Facts for Connecting Children with Nature

- Lava is the liquid expelled from the volcano.
- Volcanoes can be active, dormant or extinct.

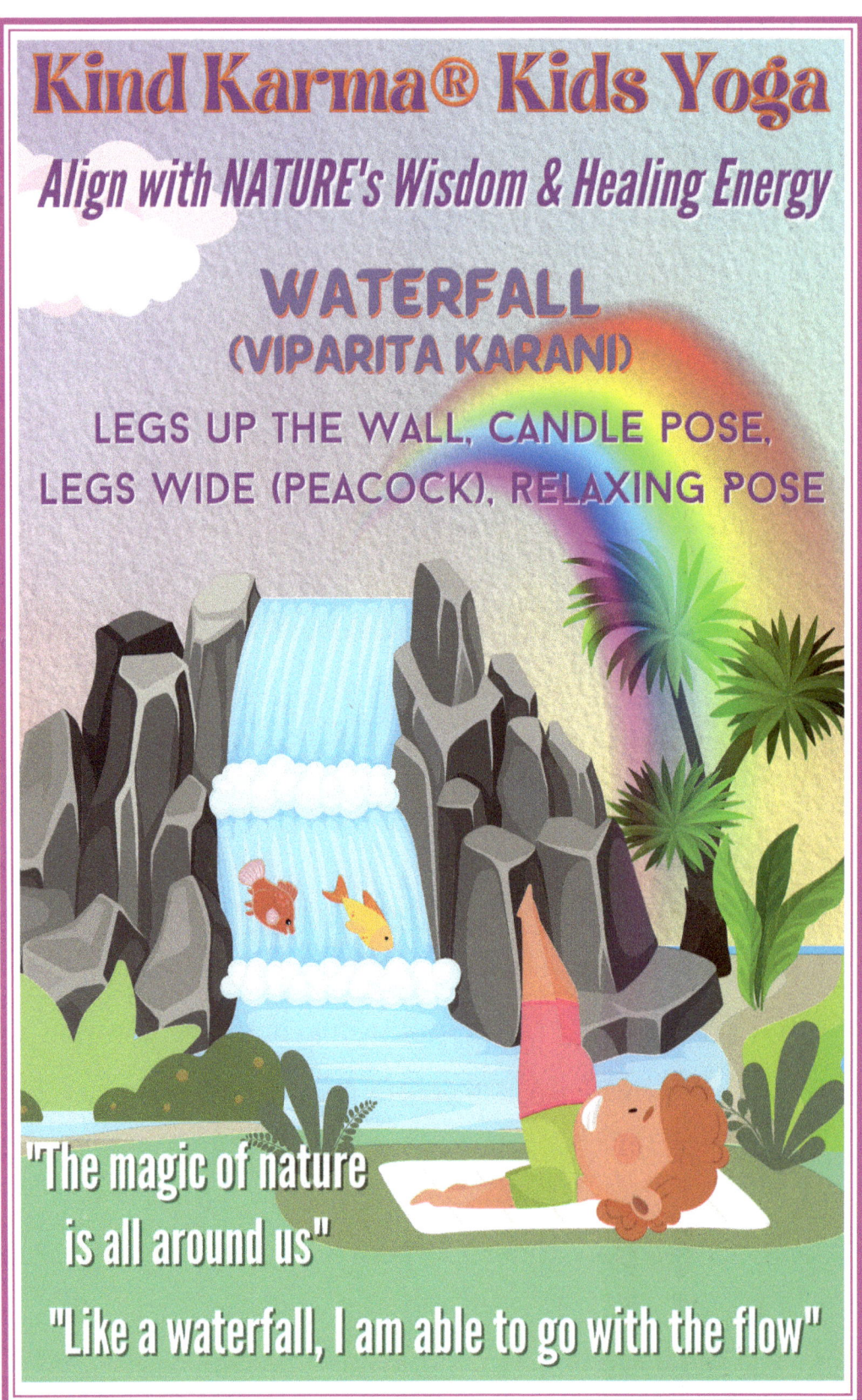

Waterfall Pose

1. Begin by laying on your back.

2. Lift your legs up towards the ceiling, and gently rest your legs against the wall. Rest your arms on the floor next to your body.

    - Your hands can be open to the sides or one hand can rest on the stomach area and the other on the heart.

3. Close your eyes, and take in long, deep breaths.

4. Hold **Waterfall Pose** for as long as desired.

5. When you are ready, roll to your side and rest there for two to three breaths. Gently sit yourself up.

Benefits

- Is a rejuvenating, mild inverted pose.
- Calms and clears the mind.
- Relaxes the body.
- Soothes the nervous system.
- Restorative for the spine, legs and feet.

Fun Facts for Connecting Children with Nature

- No two waterfalls are exactly the same, just like snowflakes and fingerprints!

- A waterfall is an area of a river or stream where the water flows over a steep or vertical drop.

Notes

SECTION II

Kind Karma Kids Yoga Animal Poses
"Tap Into The Animal Prana Power"

1. Bear Pose
2. Blissful Otter Pose
3. Buffalo Pose
4. Butterfly Pose
5. Cat Pose
6. Caterpillar Pose
7. Cobra Pose
8. Cow Pose
9. Crocodile Pose
10. Crow Pose
11. Deer Pose
12. Dog Pose
13. Eagle Pose
14. Fish Pose
15. Flamingo Pose
16. Frog Pose
17. Hedgehog Pose
18. Horse Pose
19. Jellyfish Pose
20. Kangaroo Pose
21. Lion's Breath Pose
22. Lizard Pose
23. Locust Pose
24. Monkey Leaping Pose
25. Mouse Pose
26. Pigeon Pose
27. Tiger Pose
28. Turtle Pose
29. Whale Pose
30. Wolf Pose

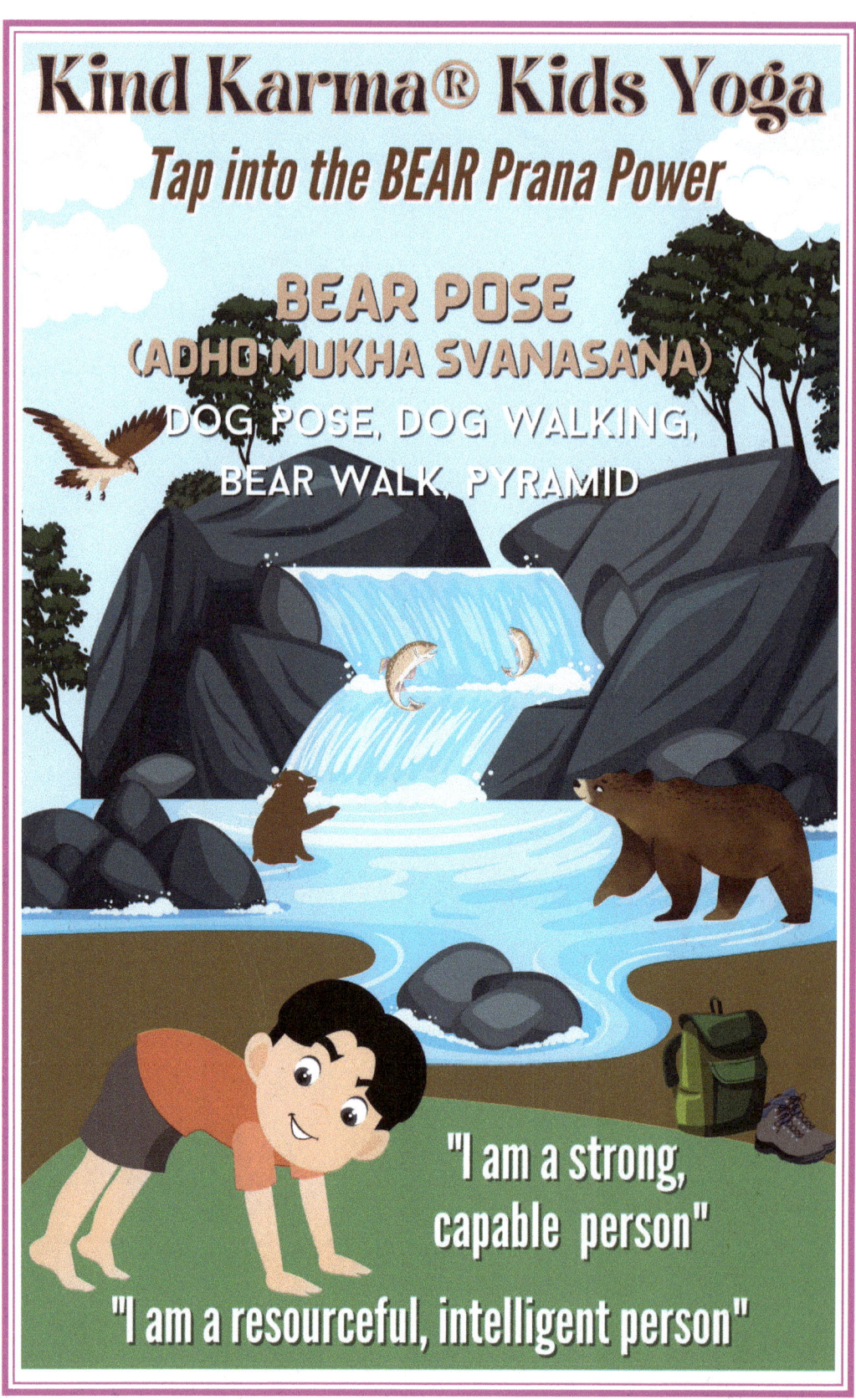

Bear Pose

1. From your hands and knees, spread your fingers out and press your hands down into the floor shoulder-width apart.

2. Curl your toes under, lift your knees off the floor and your hips up (bottom) into the air. Your body should form a triangle shape.

3. Keep your head between your upper arms.

    - You are balancing your weight on both your hands and feet.

4. If your legs feel tight, then bend your knees a little.

5. Hold Bear Pose for three to five breaths.

6. To end, lower your knees back to the floor, press your hips back toward your feet, and rest in child's pose.

Benefits

- Rejuvenating and energizing.
- Clears and calms the mind.
- Strengthens the body.
- Lengthens the spine and gives the upper and lower body a good stretch.

Corresponding Element (to embrace your *inner bear* and to help with creating *inner shaman* concepts for class lesson plans)

- Earth.

Bear Attributes (to embrace your *inner bear* and to help with creating *inner shaman* concepts for class lesson plans)

- Refer to the "Associated Animal Attributes" Table.

Corresponding Crystals for Bear Animal Prana Power

- For Personal Empowerment: Bloodstone, Carnelian, Citrine, Clear Crystal Quartz, Garnet, Hematite, Leopardskin Jasper, Smoky Quartz, Snowflake Obsidian, Turquoise.

Notes

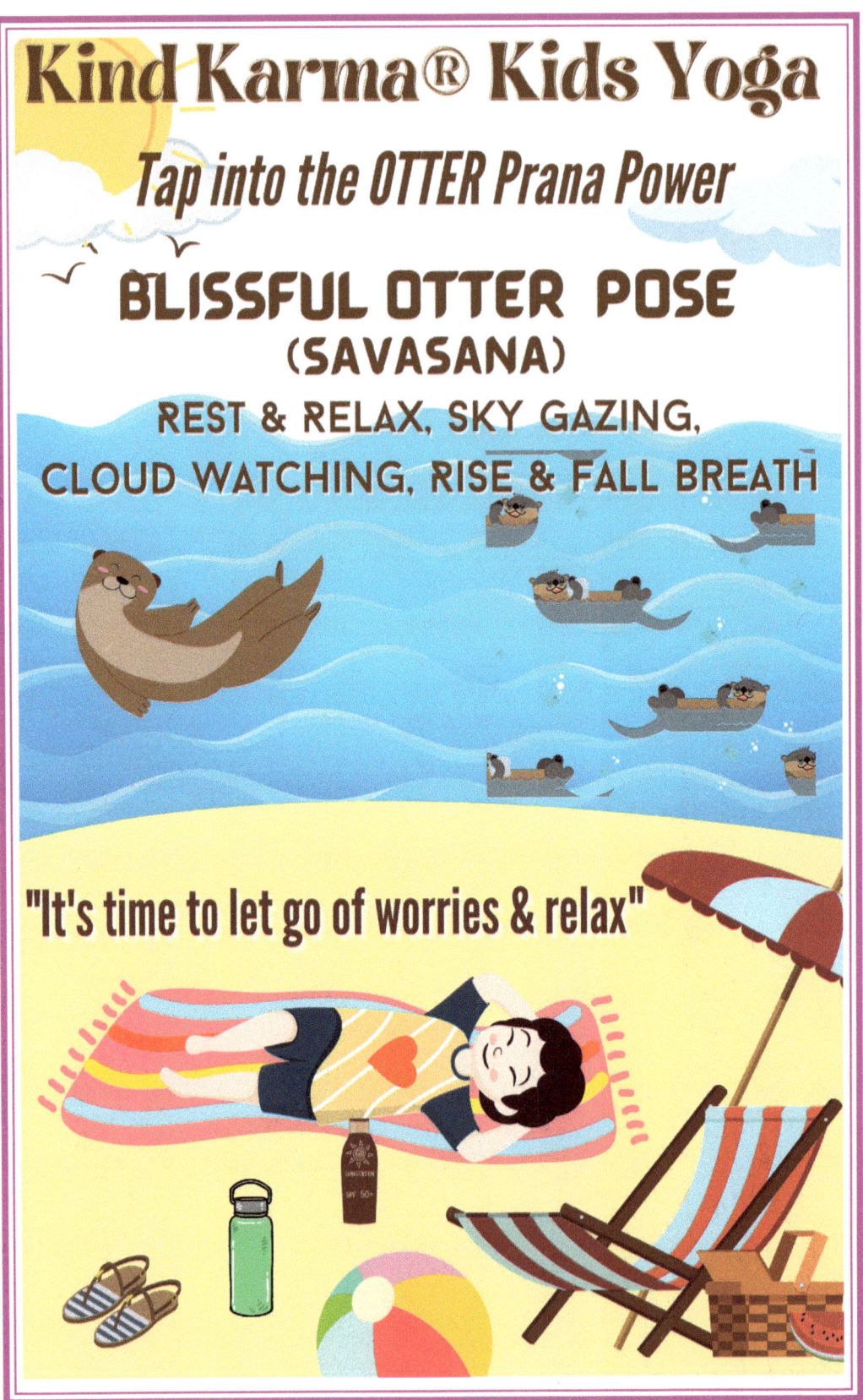

Blissful Otter Pose

1. Lie on your back with your arms and legs stretched out.
   - Allow your legs to separate and your feet to fall open.
   - Rest arms alongside your body with your palms facing up.
2. Gently close your eyes.
3. Breathe quietly and rest.
4. Remain in Blissful Otter Pose for three to five minutes.

Benefits

- Calms and clears the mind.
- Reboots and soothes the nervous system.
- Relaxes the body.
- Relieves stress and tension.

Corresponding Element (to embrace your *inner otter* and to help with creating core concepts for class lesson plans)

- Water.

Otter Attributes (to embrace your *inner otter* and to help with creating core concepts for class lesson plans)

- Refer to the "Associated Animal Attributes" Table.

Corresponding Crystals for Otter Animal Prana Power

- For Increasing Joy and Happiness: Amethyst, Carnelian, Celestite, Citrine, Crazy Lace Agate, Fluorite, Ocean Jasper, Orange Calcite, Rose Quartz, Turquoise.

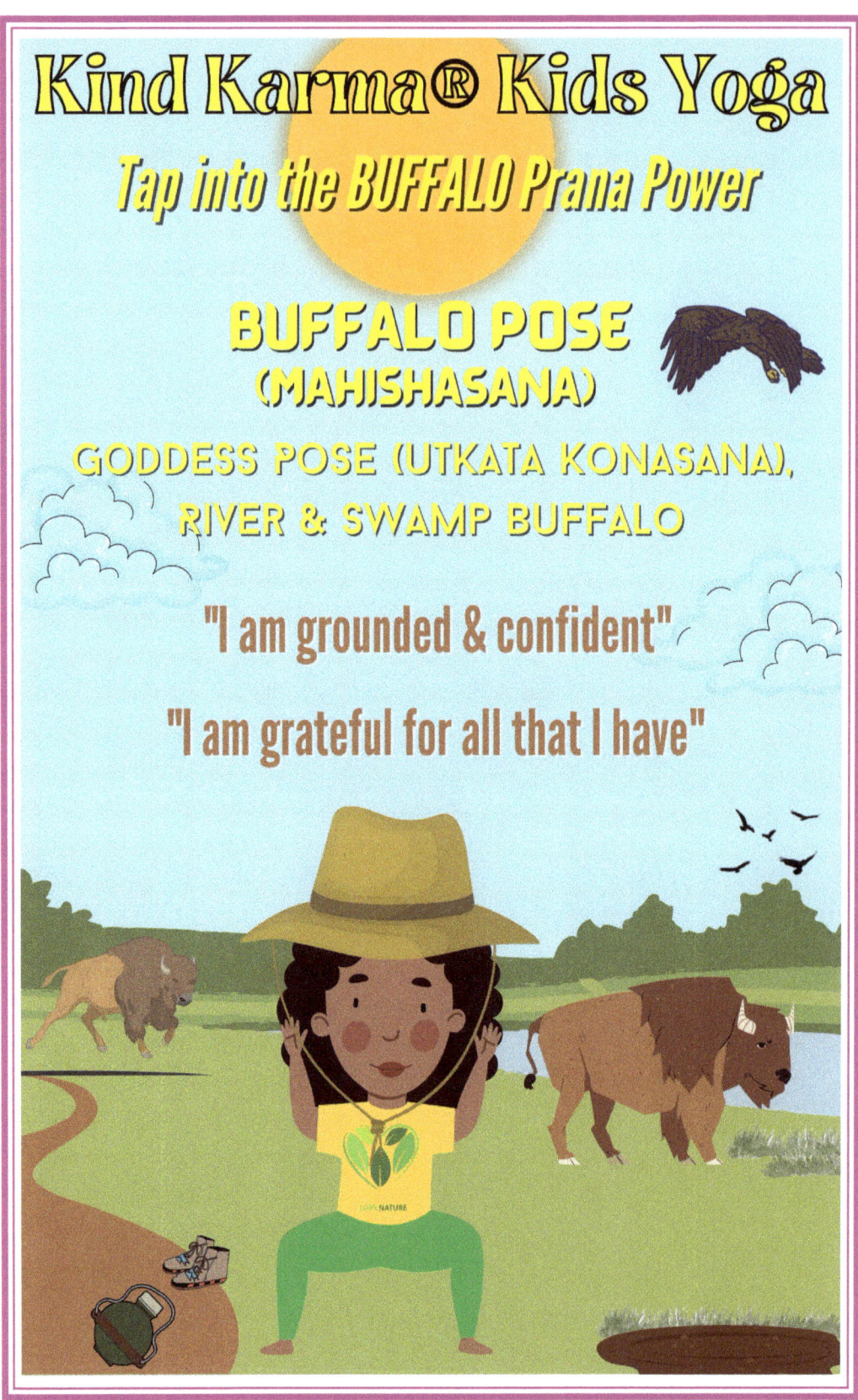

Buffalo Pose

1. Stand with your legs apart – slightly wider than shoulder distance, with your feet facing slightly outward.

2. Bend your knees 90 degrees keeping your knees pointed over feet and tailbone slightly tucked under your body.

    - Press your thighs open to keep knees from falling inward.

3. Reach your arms sideways, shoulder height, and bend your elbows 90 degrees ("cactus arms"). Face your palms forward.

    - Be sure to slide your shoulder blades downward.

4. Hold for Buffalo Pose for three to five deep breaths.

Benefits

- Strengthens the core, legs, glutes and shoulders.
- Opens and stretches the chest, upper body and inner thigh muscles.
- Lengthens the spine.
- Warms and energizes the body.
- Teaches how to ground, be strong and be present.

Corresponding Element (to embrace your *inner buffalo* and to help with creating *inner shaman* concepts for class lesson plans)

- Earth.

Buffalo Attributes (to embrace your *inner buffalo* and to help with creating *inner shaman* concepts for class lesson plans)

- Refer to the "Associated Animal Attributes" Table.

Corresponding Crystals for Buffalo Animal Prana Power

- To Attract Abundance and Success: Amazonite, Amethyst, Apache Tears, Aventurine, Citrine, Clear Quartz, Emerald, Green Aventurine, Green Jade, Malachite, Pyrite, Tiger's Eye, Turquoise.

- To Increase Gratitude and Humility: Angelite, Celestite, Chrysoprase, Green Aventurine, Malachite, Pink Opal, Rainbow Fluorite.

- To Increase Harmony and Unity: Blue Kyanite, Chalcedony, Clear Quartz, Green Tourmaline, Jade, Rose Quartz, Selenite.

Notes

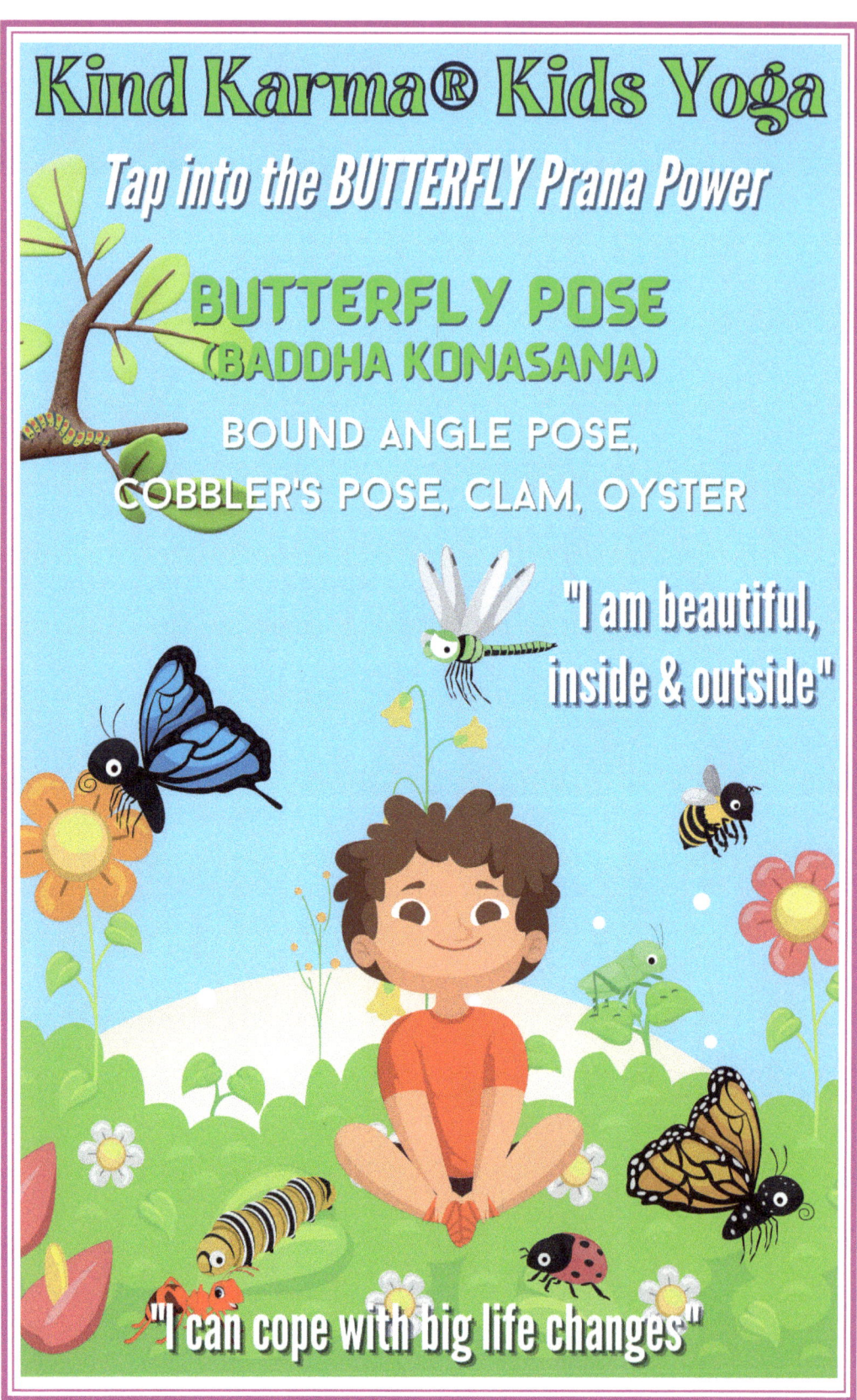

Butterfly Pose

1. Sit on the floor, or a cushion, with your spine straight and legs out in front of you.

2. Bend your knees and bring the soles of your feet together, allowing your knees to fall out to each side.

3. Wrap your hands around your ankles and gently move your knees up and down as if your legs are butterfly wings.

   - If you are uncomfortable moving the legs up and down, then just keep them still.

   - To make the pose more gentle, slowly slide your heels farther away from your body.

4. Hold Butterfly Pose for three to five breaths,

5. To end, gently bring your knees together and then stretch your legs out in front of you.

Benefits

- Stretches the groin and inner thighs.

- Release tension in the lower back, when bending forward.

- Calms the mind and releases stress.

- Moving the legs like butterfly wings helps to redirect and channel excess energy or pent up emotional energy.

Corresponding Element (to embrace your *inner butterfly* and to help with creating *inner shaman* concepts for class lesson plans)

- Air/Wind. Earth.

Butterfly Attributes (to embrace your *inner butterfly* and to help with creating *inner shaman* concepts for class lesson plans)

- Refer to the "Associated Animal Attributes" Table.

Corresponding Crystals for Butterfly Prana Power

- For Personal Transformation: Charoite, Chrysocolla, Labradorite, Malachite, Moldavite, Septarian, Shungite, Smoky Quartz, Tektite.

- To Experience the Joy of Change: Apatite, Agate, Apophyllite, Chrysoprase, Citrine, Moonstone, Rose Quartz, Septarian.

Notes

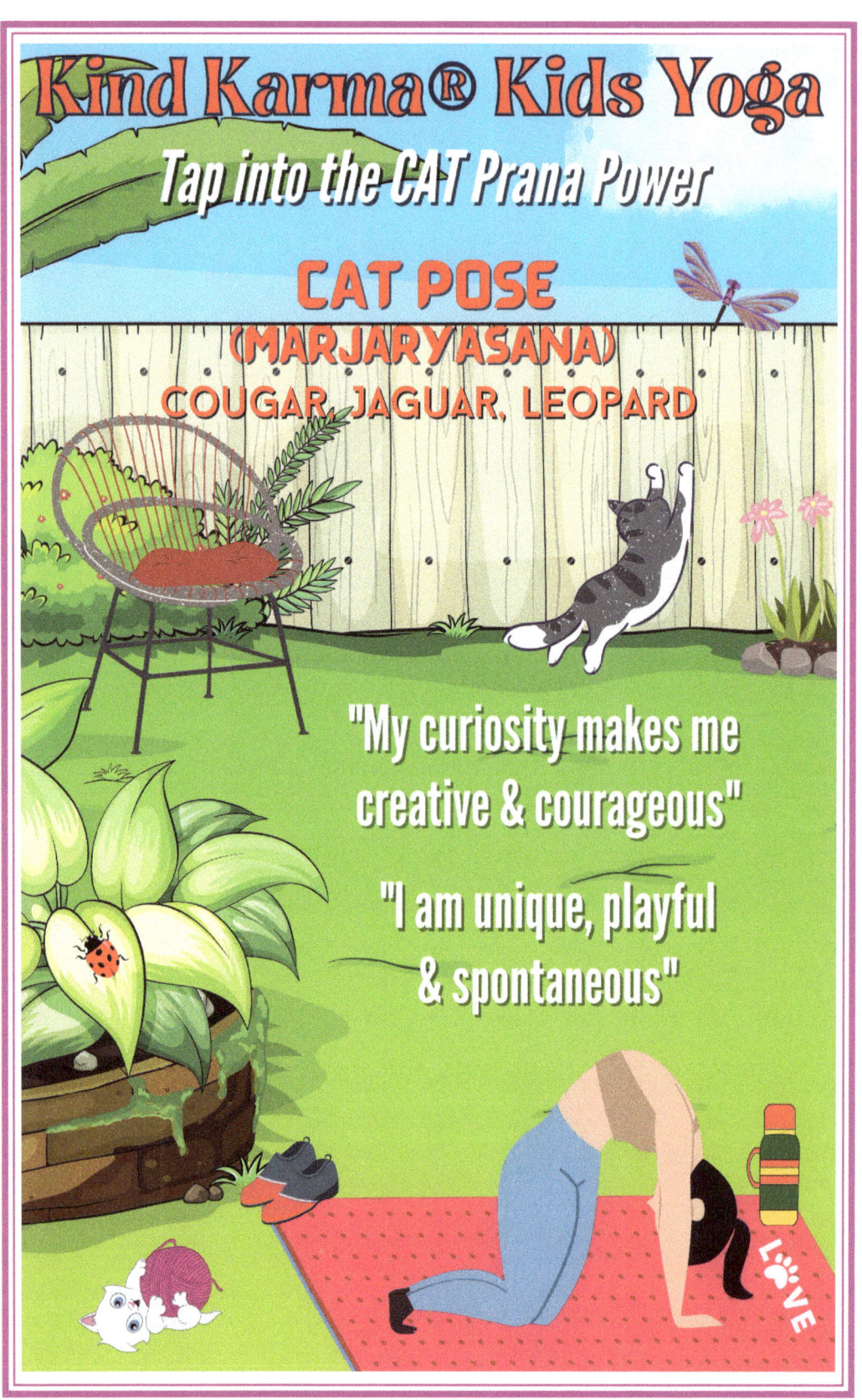

Cat Pose

1. Come onto your hands and knees in tabletop posture.

2. Spread your fingers. Check that your wrists are directly under your shoulders and your knees underneath your hips. Find your neutral spine position.

   - A neutral spine forms an S-curve: a forward curve at the neck; a backward curve in the mid-back; and another forward curve in the lower back.

3. Now exhale, gently drop your head and round your spine towards the ceiling. Try to look at your belly.

4. Tip: When rounding your spine, gently press your belly inward and tuck in your tailbone, like a cat.

5. Follow Cat Pose with Cow Pose.

6. Repeat, creating a flow between Cat and Cow Pose.

Benefits

- Relieves back and neck tension.
- Increases spine flexibility.
- Increases circulation after sitting for long periods of time.
- Strengthens the core muscles.
- Using deep breathing will release tension, stress and agitation.
- Calms and clears the mind.

Corresponding Element (to embrace your *inner cat* and to help with creating *inner shaman* concepts for class lesson plans)

- Fire.
- Spiritually, some cats can represent either an earth or air element.

Cat Attributes (to embrace your *inner cat* and to help with creating *inner shaman* concepts for class lesson plans)

- Refer to the "Associated Animal Attributes" Table.

Corresponding Crystals for Cat Prana Power

- To Develop Independence and Inner Magic (With these two particular attributes, these crystals share similar properties, hence they are grouped together): Agate, Amethyst, Aquamarine, Black Onyx, Carnelian, Garnet, Jade, Jasper, Moonstone, Nuummite, Red Tiger's Eye, Tiger's Eye.

Notes

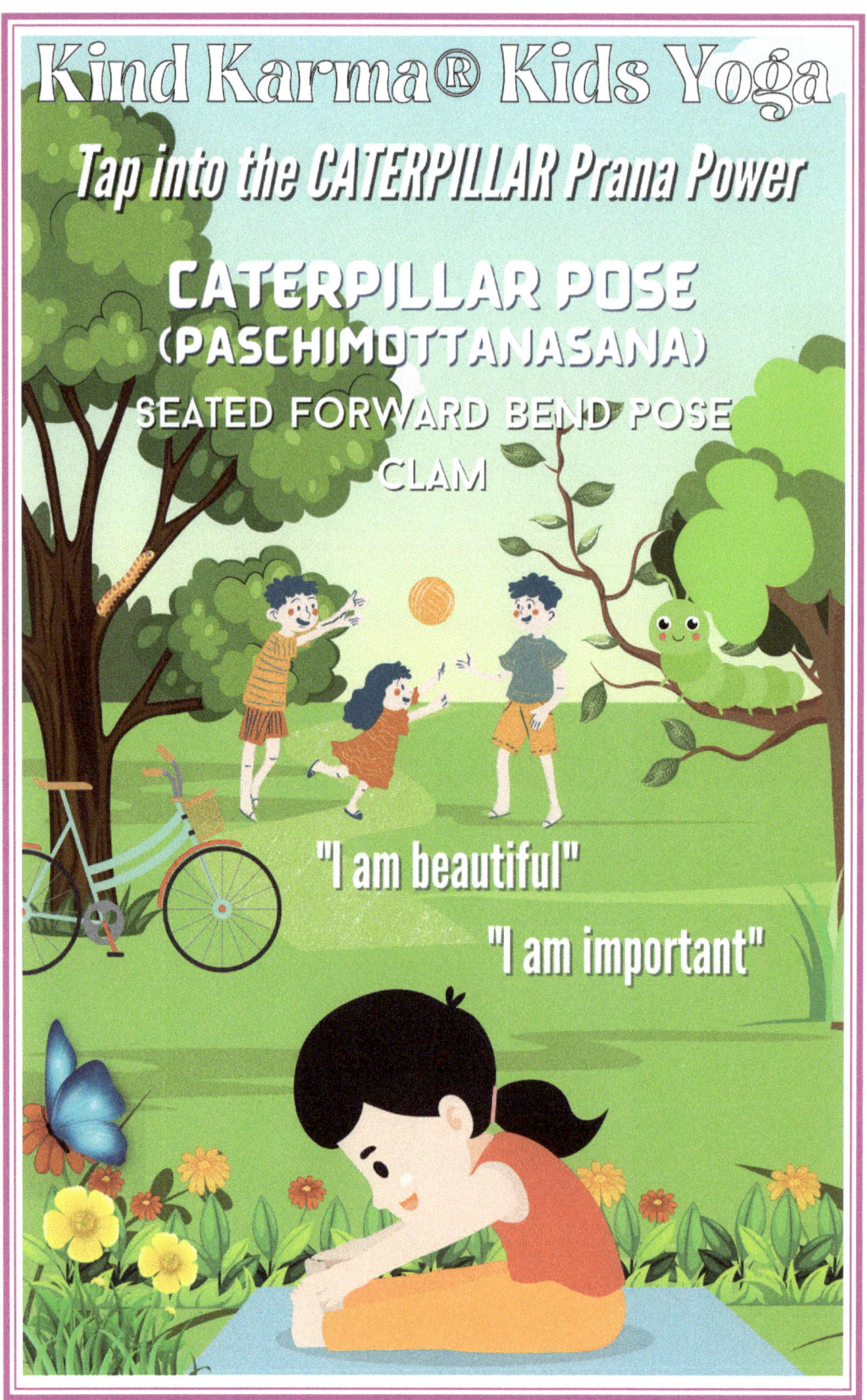

Caterpillar Pose

1. Sit on your mat or the floor, with your legs straight in front of you and your spine real tall.

2. Reach your arms up toward the ceiling, and as you do, lift your chest taller too.

3. Lean forward bringing your upper body towards your thighs.

4. Straighten your arms and reach your hands towards your feet. If you can, hold onto your toes. If this is not possible, then place your hands along the legs as far as you can reach.

5. Hold Caterpillar Pose for three to five breaths.

6. To end, slowly return to sitting upright.

Benefits

- Stretches the legs and back.
- Calms and clears the mind.
- Reduces stress and restlessness.
- Very grounding.
- Allows for introspection.

Corresponding Element (to embrace your *inner caterpillar* and to help with creating *inner shaman* concepts for class lesson plans)

- Earth.
- Air (Relating to the potential of turning into a butterfly).

Caterpillar Attributes (to embrace your *inner caterpillar* and to help with creating *inner shaman* concepts for class lesson plans)

- Refer to the "Associated Animal Attributes" Table.

Corresponding Crystals for Caterpillar Prana Power

- For Personal Transformation: Amethyst, Charoite, Chrysocolla, Labradorite, Malachite, Moldavite, Rutilated Quartz, Shungite, Smoky Quartz, Tektite.
- To Increase Patience: Amber, Aventurine, Blue Lace Agate, Chrysoprase, Dumortierite, Emerald, Green Jade, Howlite, Moss Agate, Septarian.

Notes

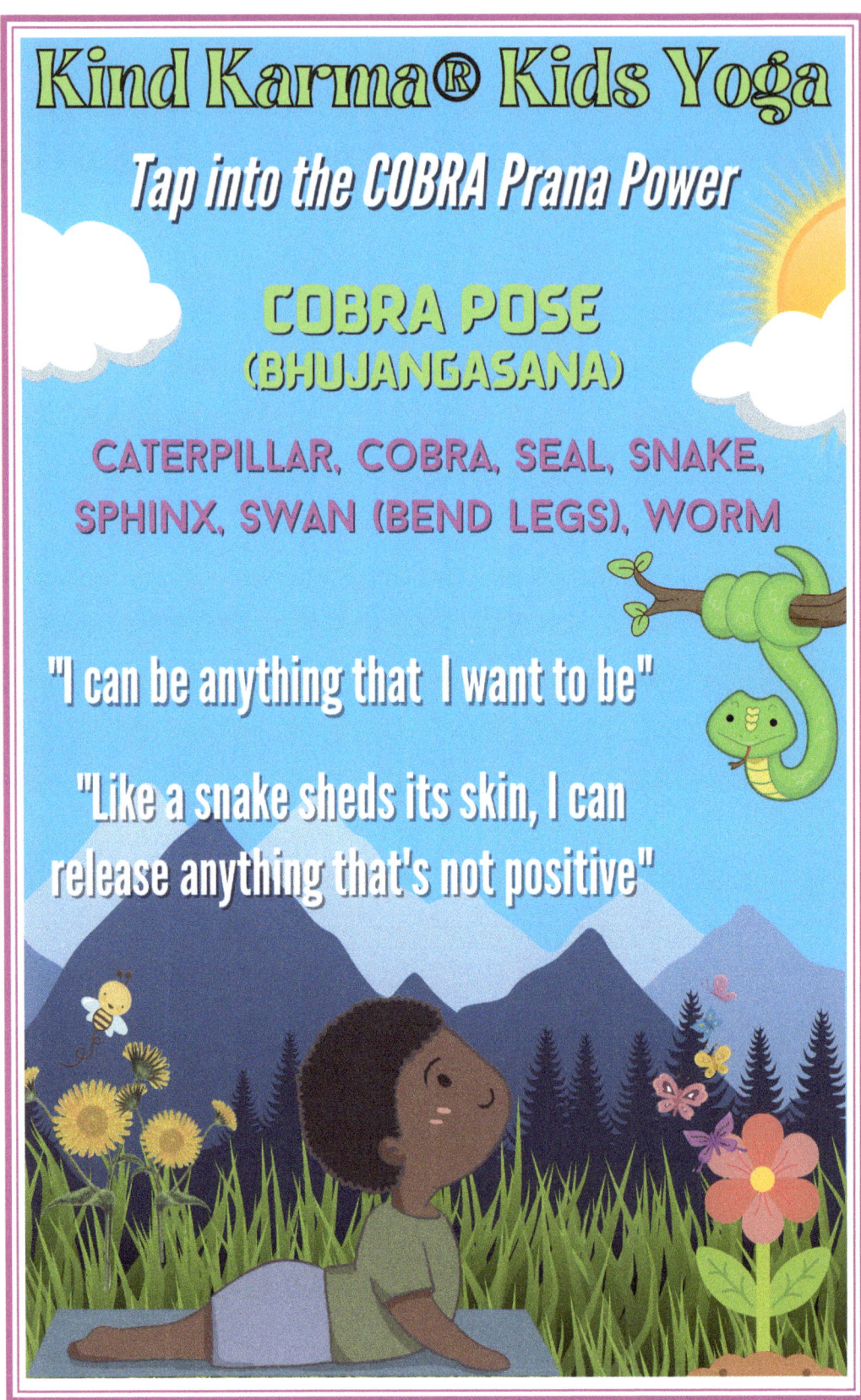

Cobra Pose

1. Lie on your belly with your legs straight out behind you. Keep your legs and feet slightly apart.

   - Tip: Energize your lower body by pressing your thighs and the tops of your feet against the ground.

   - Tip: Firm your thighs and glutes.

2. Place your palms by your shoulders and gently draw your shoulder blades together down your back.

3. Inhale, and press your hands into the floor and gently lift your head, chest, and shoulders off the floor. Straighten your arms as far as feels comfortable.

4. Look in front of you to make sure that your neck is in proper alignment.

5. Hold Cobra Pose for three to five breaths.

6. Exhale and lower yourself back to the ground. For a couple of breaths, allow your lower back to relax.

Benefits

- Stretches, lengthens and warms up the spine.
- Stretches the chest, shoulders and belly.
- Strengthens the spine, back muscles, chest and arms.
- Good corrective stretch after sitting.
- Awakens the body and elevates the mood.

Corresponding Element (to embrace your *inner cobra* and to help with creating *inner shaman* concepts for class lesson plans)

- Earth.
- Fire.

Cobra Attributes (to embrace your *inner cobra* and to help with creating *inner shaman* concepts for class lesson plans)

- Refer to the "Associated Animal Attributes" Table.

Corresponding Crystals for Cobra Prana Power

- For Inner Growth: Amazonite, Aquamarine, Aventurine, Bloodstone, Blue Lace Agate, Chrysocolla, Citrine, Moss Agate, Onyx, Smoky Quartz.

- For Personal Transformation: Amethyst, Charoite, Chrysocolla, Labradorite, Malachite, Moldavite, Rutilated Quartz, Shungite, Smoky Quartz, Tektite.

Notes

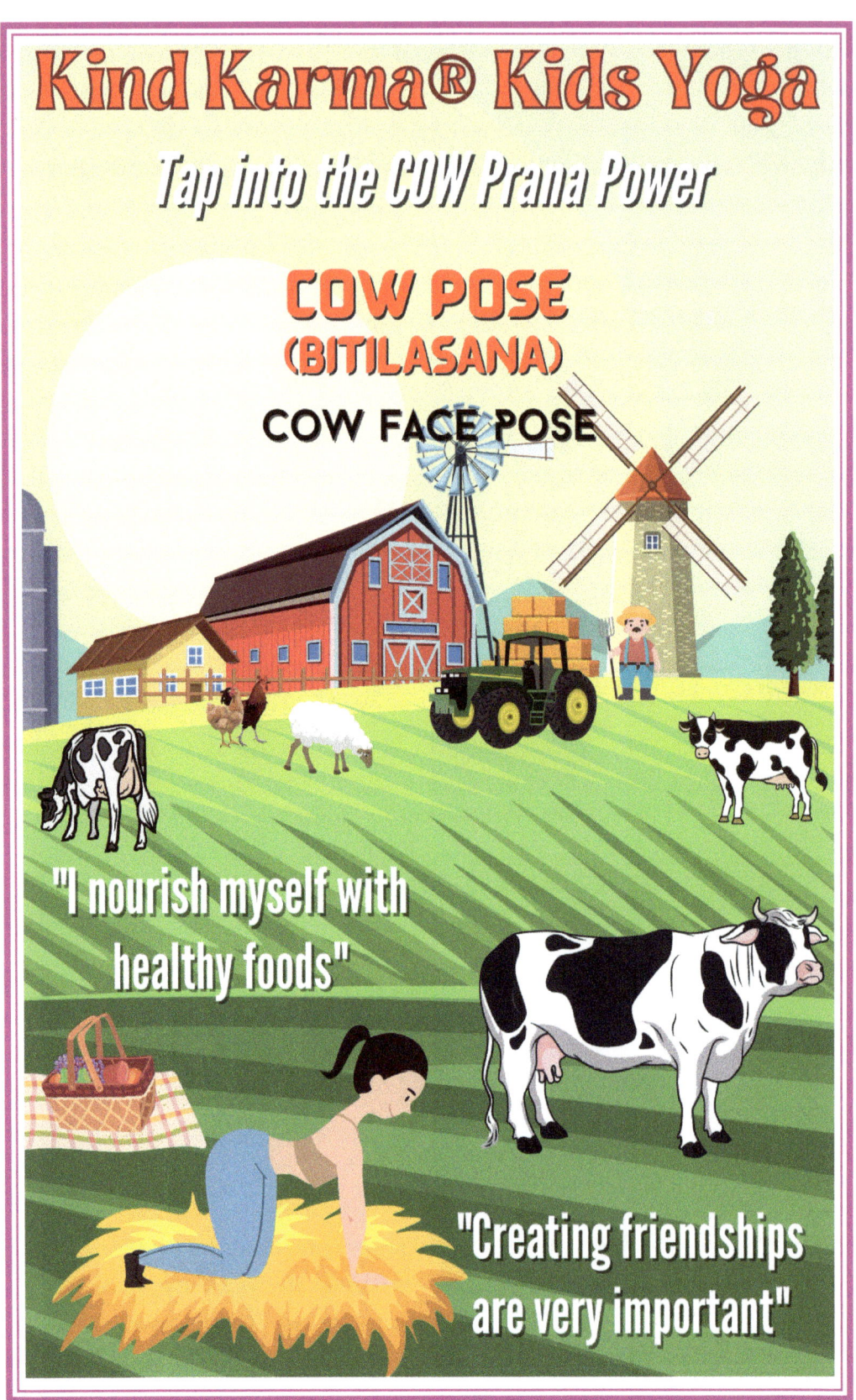

Cow Pose

1. Come onto your hands and knees in tabletop posture.

2. Spread your fingers. Check that your wrists are directly under your shoulders and your knees underneath your hips. Find your neutral spine position.

   - A neutral spine forms an S-curve: a forward curve at the neck; a backward curve in the mid-back; and another forward curve in the lower back.

3. Now inhale and look up to the ceiling, and allow your belly to sink towards the floor.

   - Tip: Lift your chest and tailbone toward the ceiling.

   - Tip: Allow your belly to relax towards the floor.

4. Follow Cow Pose with Cat Pose.

5. Repeat, creating a flow between Cat and Cow Pose.

Benefits

- Stretches, lengthens and warms up the spine.
- Stretches the chest, shoulders and belly.
- Strengthens the spine, back muscles, chest and arms.
- Good corrective stretch after sitting.
- Awakens the body and elevates the mood.

Corresponding Element (to embrace your *inner cow* and to help with creating *inner shaman* concepts for class lesson plans)

- Earth.

Cow Attributes (to embrace your *inner cow* and to help with creating *inner shaman* concepts for class lesson plans)

- Refer to the "Associated Animal Attributes" Table.

Corresponding Crystals for Cow Prana Power

- For Calming and Stress Relief: Amethyst, Angelite, Aquamarine, Black Tourmaline, Blue Lace Agate, Celestite, Howlite, Lepidolite, Morganite, Moss Agate, Rose Quartz, Selenite.

Notes

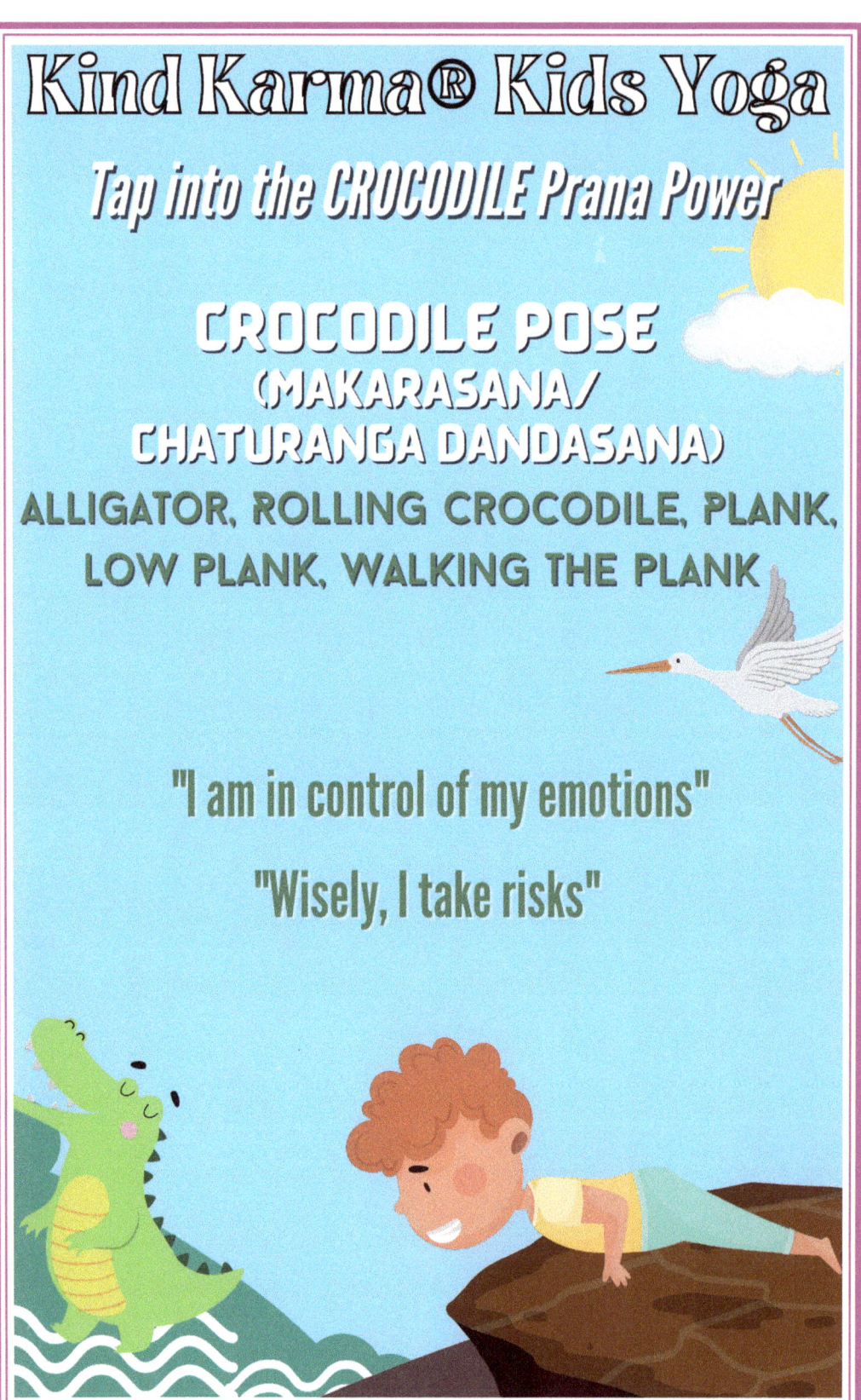

Crocodile Pose

1. From all fours, walk your hands forward and come into Plank Pose with your hands under your shoulders.

2. Straighten your legs, until they are a few inches above the ground and parallel to it, with your toes turned inwards.

3. On an exhalation, bend your elbows until your shoulders are at the same height as your elbows.

   - Tip: If this is too challenging, lower your knees to the floor for support as you lower your upper body downward.

   - Tip: Lower yourself only as far as you comfortably can.

4. Hold Crocodile Pose for three to five breaths.

5. Exhale as you come up (push up) back into Plank Pose.

6. To end, come onto your hands and knees.

Benefits

- Increases overall body strength and tone.
- Strengthens the core, back and arm muscles.
- Builds flexibility and strength in the wrists.
- Improves posture.
- Invigorates the body and mind.
- Teaches how to navigate through challenges.

Corresponding Element (to embrace your *inner crocodile* and to help with creating *inner shaman* concepts for class lesson plans)

- Water.
- Earth.

Crocodile Attributes (to embrace your *inner crocodile* and to help with creating *inner shaman* concepts for class lesson plans)

- Refer to the "Associated Animal Attributes" Table.

Corresponding Crystals for Crocodile Prana Power

- To Find your Courage and Build Confidence: Amazonite, Aquamarine, Black Tourmaline, Carnelian, Citrine, Dolomite, Garnet, Orange Calcite, Red Jasper, Rose Quartz, Septarian, Spirit Quartz, Sodalite, Sunstone, Tiger's Eye.

Notes

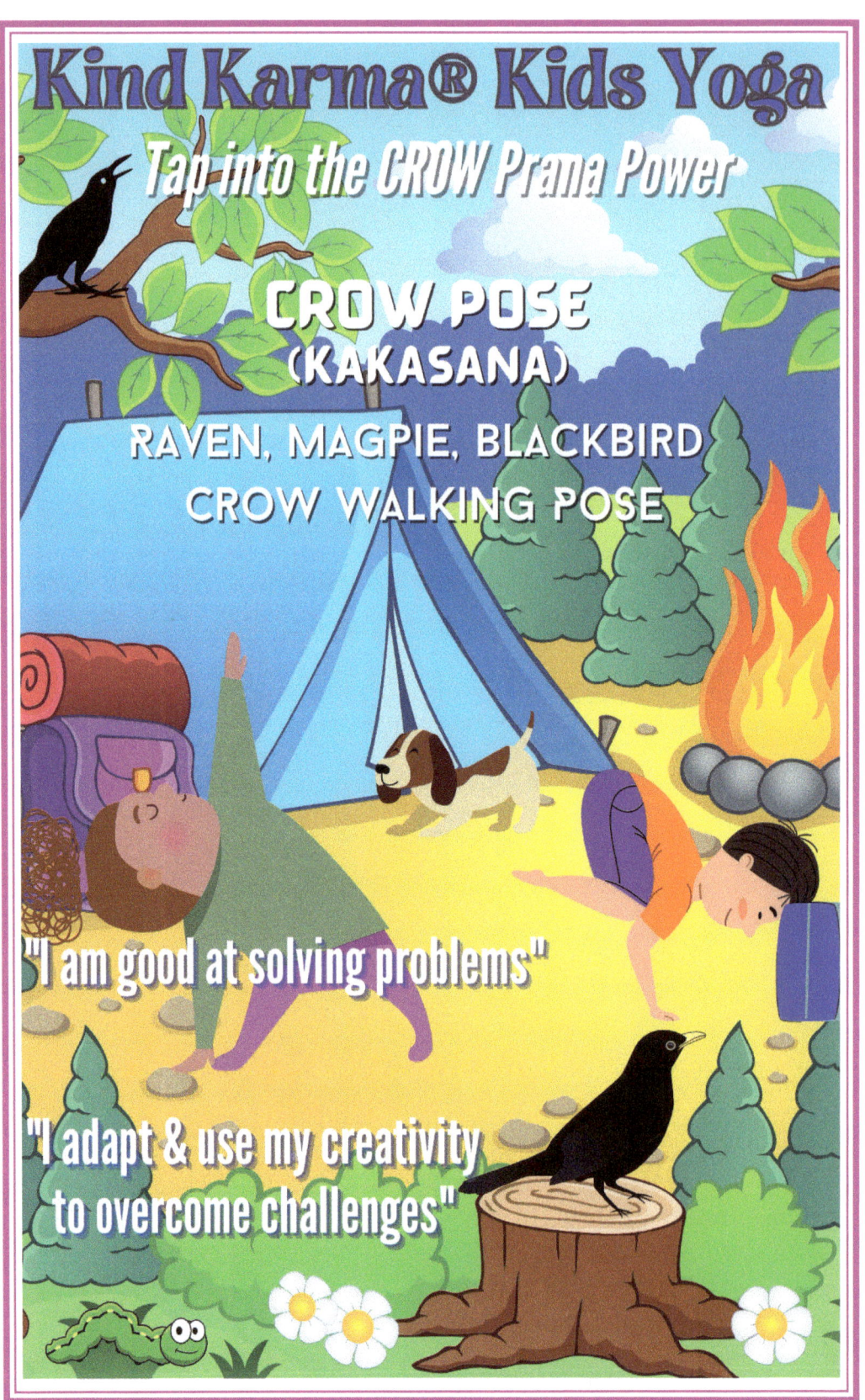

Crow Pose

1. Lower yourself into a squatting position with your arms between your legs.

2. Place your hands on your mat in front of you, shoulder-width apart.

3. Bend your elbows, and lean forward to touch your shins to your upper arms.

4. Lift up on the balls of your feet, and continue to lean forward until your feet leave the floor and you are balancing on your hands.

    - Tip: To increase stability, look slightly ahead at the floor, and lift one foot off the ground then the other.

    - Tip: Firm your abdominal muscles.

5. Hold Crow Pose for three to five breaths (or as long as you comfortably can), then slowly return to your mat in a squatting position.

Benefits

- Increases overall body strength, especially the upper body.
- Strengthens and tones the core.
- Improves body control.
- Builds confidence.
- Develops the ability to focus.
- Invigorates the body and mind.
- Teaches how to navigate through challenges.

Corresponding Element (to embrace your *inner crow* and to help with creating *inner shaman* concepts for class lesson plans)

- Air/Wind.

Crow Attributes (to embrace your *inner crow* and to help with creating *inner shaman* concepts for class lesson plans)

- Refer to the "Associated Animal Attributes" Table.

Corresponding Crystals for Crow Prana Power

- To Improve Focus and Mental Clarity: Amethyst, Apatite, Black Tourmaline, Clear Quartz, Citrine, Fluorite, Hematite, Lapis Lazuli, Onyx, Prehnite, Shungite, Sodalite, Tiger's Eye.

Notes

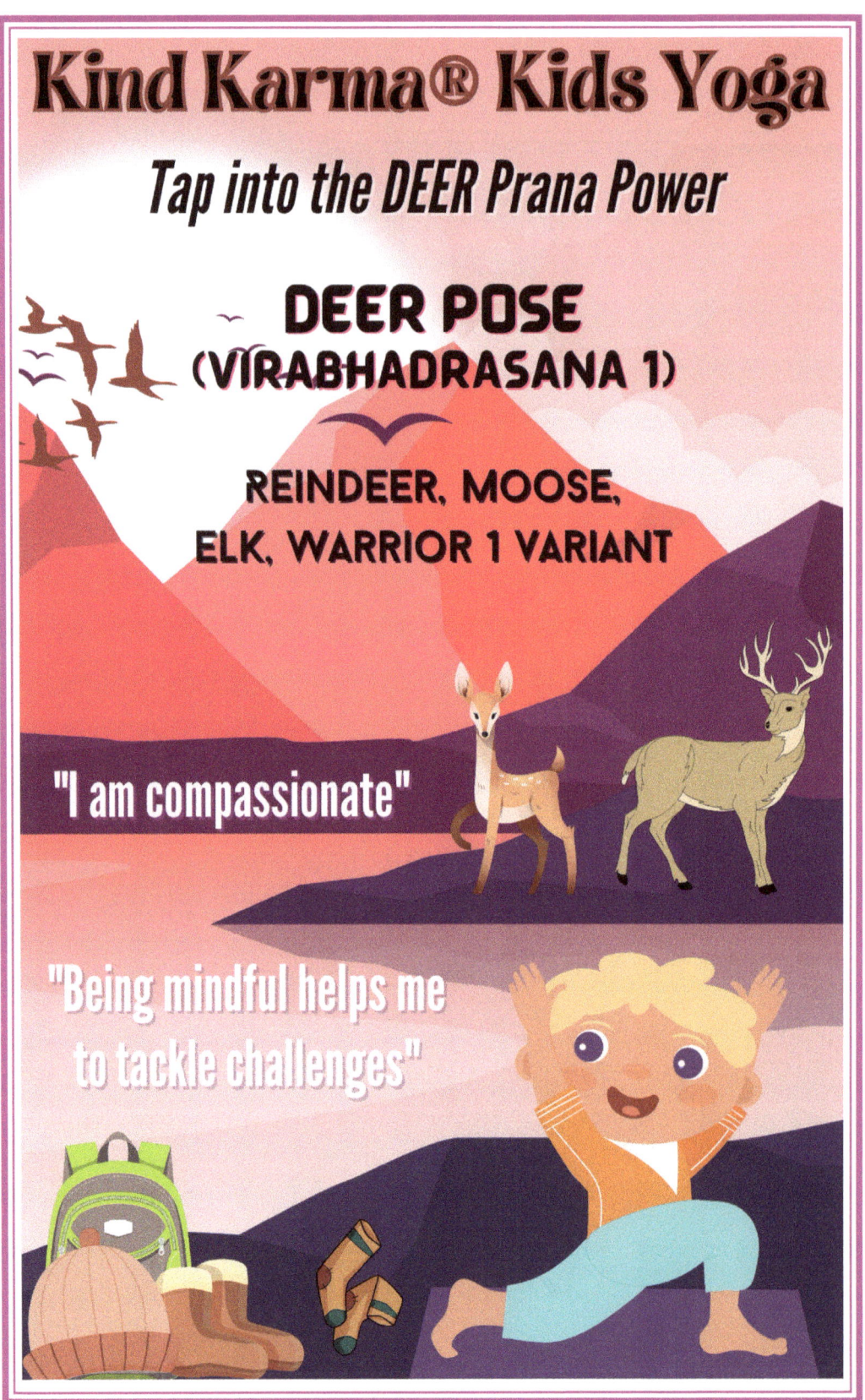

Deer Pose

1. From Mountain Pose, take a big step backward with one foot, leaving the other foot in place.

2. Take a deep breath in. As you breathe out, bend your front knee so that it comes directly over your ankle in a straight line.

3. Press your weight through your back heel. Make sure your heel remains planted on the ground.

   - Tip: If it's difficult to balance, take a wider stance.

4. Take a deep breath and reach your arms upward. Spread your fingers apart like deer antlers.

   - Tip: Feel strong and powerful.

5. Hold this Deer Pose for three to five breaths, then bring your legs together, returning to Mountain Pose.

6. Repeat with the other leg forward.

Benefits

- Strengthens the legs and core muscles.
- Improves balance.
- Enhances body awareness.
- Stretches and opens the hips.
- Increases stamina and energizes the entire body.
- Improves focus.
- Inspires confidence.

Corresponding Element (to embrace your *inner deer* and to help with creating *inner shaman* concepts for class lesson plans)

- Earth.

- Air (The antelope or deer is associated with the Heart Chakra, lightness and grace).

Deer Attributes (to embrace your *inner deer* and to help with creating *inner shaman* concepts for class lesson plans)

- Refer to the "Associated Animal Attributes" Table.

Corresponding Crystals for Deer Prana Power

- To Nurture Compassion: Amazonite, Aquamarine, Blue Aragonite, Emerald, Green Jade, Kunzite, Lapis Lazuli, Malachite, Mangano Calcite, Morganite, Pink Calcite, Pink Tourmaline, Prehnite, Rhodonite, Rose Quartz.

Notes

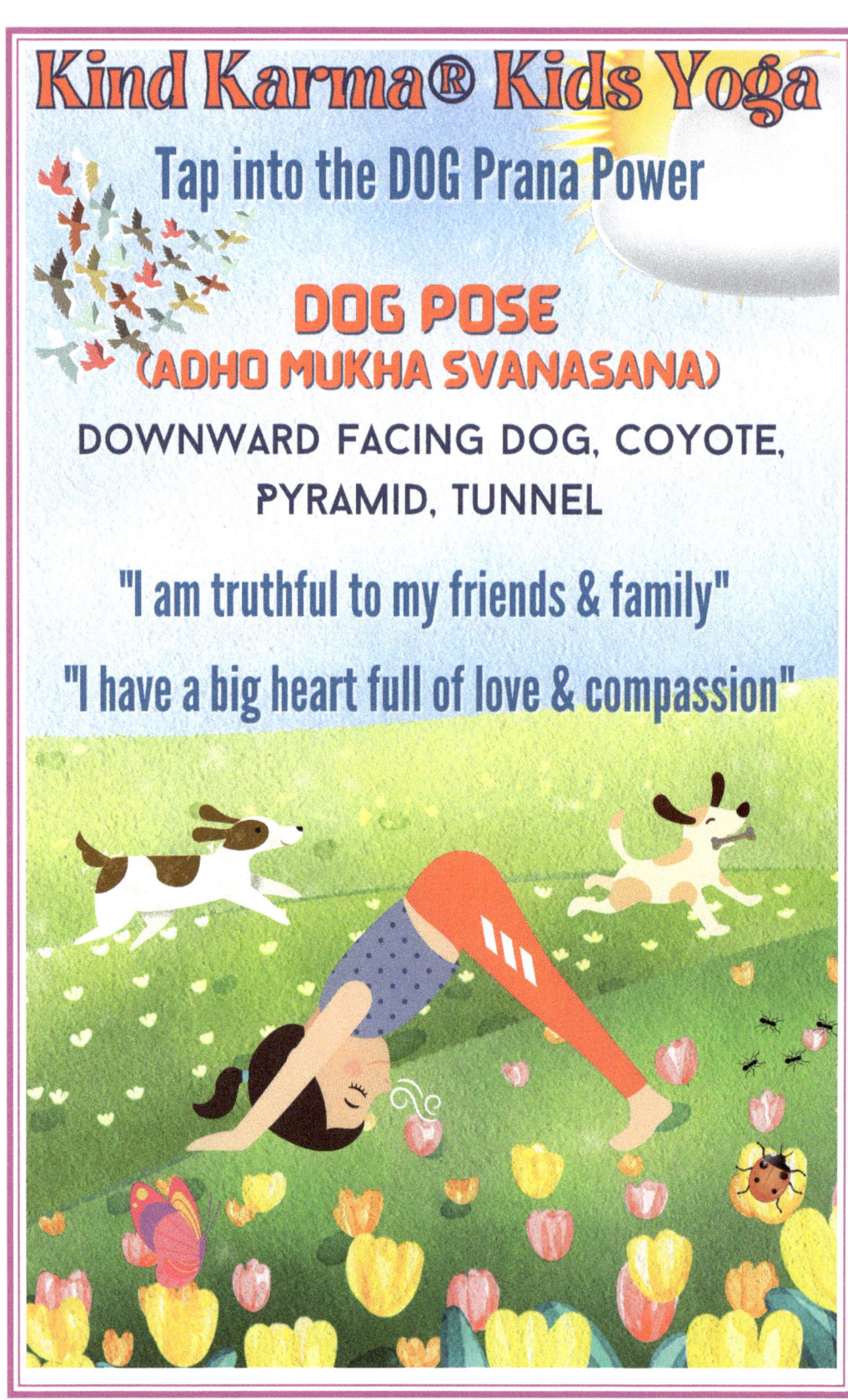

Dog Pose

1. Begin on all fours, knees under hips, hands under shoulders.
2. Spread your fingers wide and press your hands down into the floor.
3. Curl your toes under, straighten your knees and lift your hips up towards the sky, forming a pyramid shape.
   - Tip: Keep your head between your upper arms.
   - Tip: If you feel tightness down the back of your legs, bend your knees a little.
4. Hold Dog Pose for three to five breaths.
5. To come out of it, lower your knees to the floor.

Benefits

- Strengthens the entire body.
- Improves flexibility.
- Both calming and invigorating for the body and mind.
- Relieves stress.
- Nurtures a child's imagination and creativity.
- Inspires playfulness.

Corresponding Element (to embrace your *inner dog* and to help with creating *inner shaman* concepts for class lesson plans)

- Earth.

Dog Attributes (to embrace your *inner dog* and to help with creating *inner shaman* concepts for class lesson plans)

- Refer to the "Associated Animal Attributes" Table.

Corresponding Crystals for Dog Prana Power

- To Nurture Love and Compassion: Amazonite, Amethyst, Aquamarine, Aventurine, Blue Aragonite, Chrysocolla, Emerald, Green Jade, Kunzite, Lapis Lazuli, Malachite, Mangano Calcite, Moonstone, Morganite, Obsidian, Pink Calcite, Pink Tourmaline, Prehnite, Rhodochrosite, Rose Quartz, Ruby.

Notes

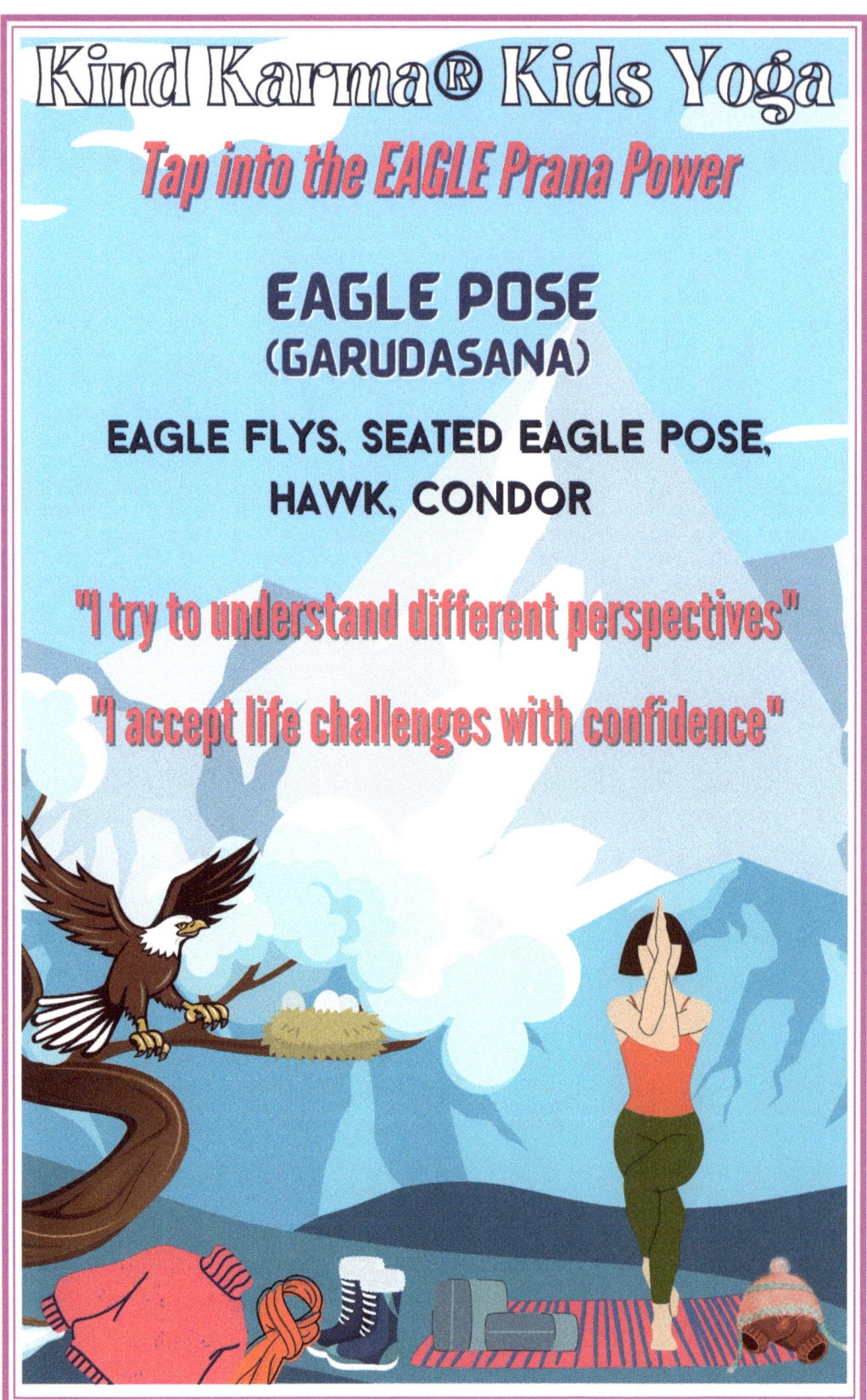

Eagle Pose

1. Begin in Mountain Pose, with your feet close together.

2. Extend your arms in front of your body.

3. Now cross your arms at the center of your chest, placing elbow over elbow, making an "X".

4. Entwine your arms together and give yourself a hug.

5. Try to place your palms together (prayer position), or as close as you can down your forearm or hand. Keep your arms lifted at chest level.

    - Tip: A good practice is just using the arms, and not crossing the legs until the next class or practice.

6. Now, bend your knees and cross one leg over the thigh and wrap it behind the calf.

    - Tip: A good practice is just using the legs, and not crossing the legs until the next class or practice.

7. Hold Eagle Pose for three to five breaths. Build up gradually.

8. To end, unwind your legs and arms, give your arms and legs a good releasing shake, and repeat on the other side.

Benefits

- Entwining and twisting the arms and legs invigorates the brain and nervous system.

- Increases strength, and improves flexibility and balance.

- Involves the entire body, including the core muscles.

- Increases concentration and focus.
- Develops body awareness and encourages proprioceptive input.

Corresponding Element (to embrace your *inner eagle* and to help with creating *inner shaman* concepts for class lesson plans)

- Air.

Eagle Attributes (to embrace your *inner eagle* and to help with creating *inner shaman* concepts for class lesson plans)

- Refer to the "Associated Animal Attributes" Table.

Corresponding Crystals for Eagle Prana Power

To Increase Confidence and Courage: Amazonite, Black Tourmaline, Carnelian, Citrine, Dolomite, Garnet, Orange Calcite, Red Jasper, Rose Quartz, Septarian, Spirit Quartz, Sodalite, Sunstone, Tiger's Eye.

Notes

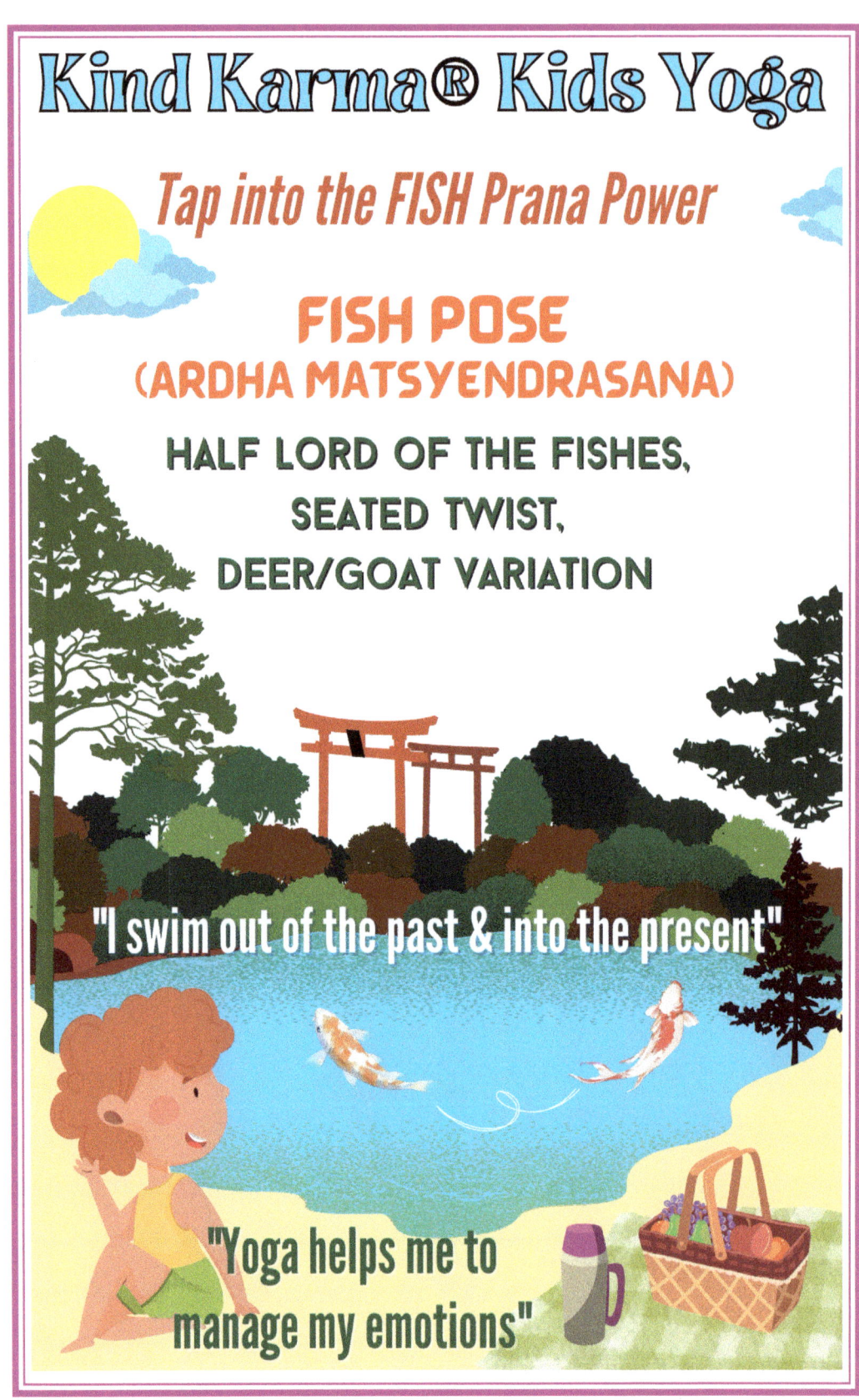

Fish Pose

1. Begin sitting on your heels in Thunderbolt Pose.

2. Shift your hips to the left so that you're sitting on the floor to the left of your feet.

3. Cross your right foot just outside of your left knee.

   - Tip: Be sure to keep the right foot flat on the floor.

4. Bring your right hand to the floor a few inches behind you.

   - Tip: Like a kickstand, use your hand to push into the ground to help straighten your spine.

5. Inhale and reach your left hand toward the sky. Exhale and bend your left arm, using your elbow like a lever against your right knee. Gaze over your right shoulder.

   - Tip: Take extra care to avoid neck pain by not turning or stretching your neck too far.

6. Remain in Fish Pose for three to five breaths.

7. To end, gently unwind and repeat to the other side.

Benefits

- Lengthens and energizes the spine.
- Increases hip and spine flexibility.
- Provides a good stretch for the outer hips and thighs.
- Tones and strengthens the abdominal and oblique muscles.
- Opens the neck, chest and shoulders.

- Increases posture awareness.
- Relieves tension, stiffness and tightness along the spine, neck and upper body.

Corresponding Element (to embrace your *inner fish* and to help with creating *inner shaman* concepts for class lesson plans)

- Water.

Fish Attributes (to embrace your *inner fish* and to help with creating *inner shaman* concepts for class lesson plans)

- Refer to the "Associated Animal Attributes" Table.

Corresponding Crystals for Fish Prana Power

To Navigate through Challenging Times and Difficult Situations: Amazonite, Bloodstone, Bronzite, Bumblebee Jasper, Citrine, Hematite, Labradorite, Pietersite, Rainbow Moonstone, Red Jasper, Rose Quartz, Shungite, Tiger's Eye, Turquoise, Unakite.

Notes

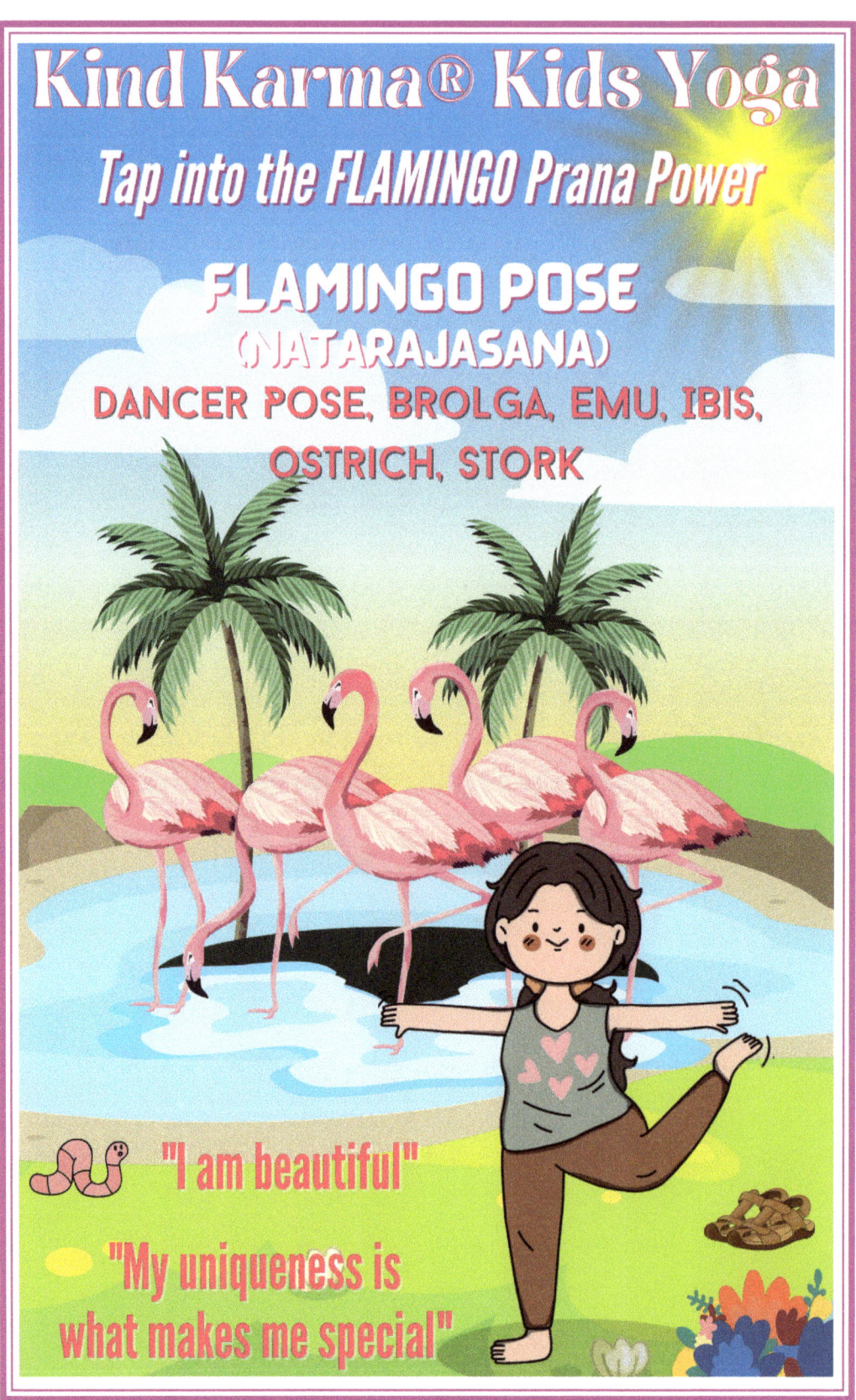

Flamingo Pose

1. Begin standing tall in Mountain Pose.

2. Shift your weight to your right foot and reach back with your left hand to hold onto your left foot or ankle.

3. Keep your body facing forward and upright and reach your free hand out (right hand).

   - Tip: To ease balance concerns, gaze out in front of you.

4. Hold Dancer Pose for three to five breaths.

5. To end, carefully release your left foot and return back to Mountain Pose. Repeat on your opposite side.

Benefits

- Improves balance.
- Lengthens and energizes the spine.
- Strengthens your legs and core.
- Stretches your chest, hips and thighs.
- Increasing focus and concentration.
- Builds confidence.

Corresponding Element (to embrace your *inner flamingo* and to help with creating *inner shaman* concepts for class lesson plans)

- Water.
- Air.

Flamingo Attributes (to embrace your *inner flamingo* and to help with creating *inner shaman* concepts for class lesson plans)

- Refer to the "Associated Animal Attributes" Table.

Corresponding Crystals for Flamingo Prana Power

For Balance and Inner Peace: Agate, Amethyst, Blue Chalcedony, Blue Lace Agate, Clear Quartz, Diopside, Fluorite, Green Jade, Green Tourmaline, Larimar, Lepidolite, Pink Calcite, Rose Quartz, Selenite, Unakite.

Notes

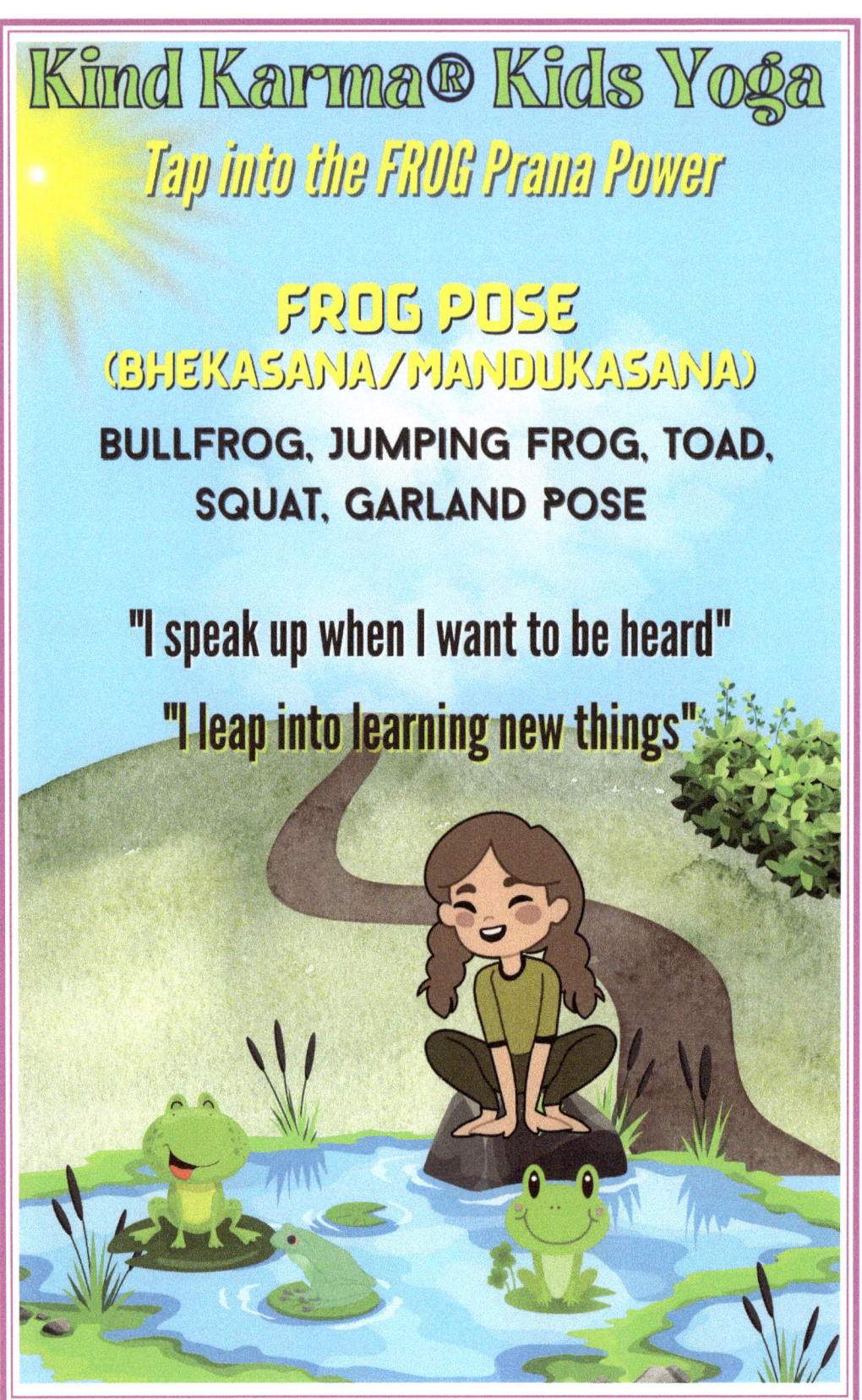

Frog Pose

1. Stand tall in Mountain Pose.

2. Move your feet hip-width apart, with your toes slightly pointed outward.

3. Bend your knees and squat, placing your hands or fingertips, on the floor between your feet.

4. Do a few soft bounces to prepare for jumping.

5. Now, jump up as you reach your hands above your head towards the sky.

    - Tip: Using the hands to push away from the ground will help to jump higher.

6. If comfortable, repeat the Frog Pose with jumping two to three more times.

Benefits

- Strengthens the shoulders, hips, legs, calves and core muscles.
- Activates the muscles of the ankles and feet.
- Improves flexibility of spine, legs, hips, knees and ankles.
- Increases proper posture awareness.
- A great wake-up movement.
- Releases stress and anxiousness.
- Inspires interactive play.

Corresponding Element (to embrace your *inner frog* and to help with creating *inner shaman* concepts for class lesson plans)

- Water.
- Earth.

Frog Attributes (to embrace your *inner frog* and to help with creating *inner shaman* concepts for class lesson plans)

- Refer to the "Associated Animal Attributes" Table.

Corresponding Crystals for Frog Prana Power

- To Find Your Voice and For Communication: Amazonite, Amethyst, Aquamarine, Azurite, Blue Lace Agate, Blue Kyanite, Carnelian, Chrysocolla, Citrine, Clear Quartz, Lapis Lazuli, Smoky Quartz, Sodalite.

Notes

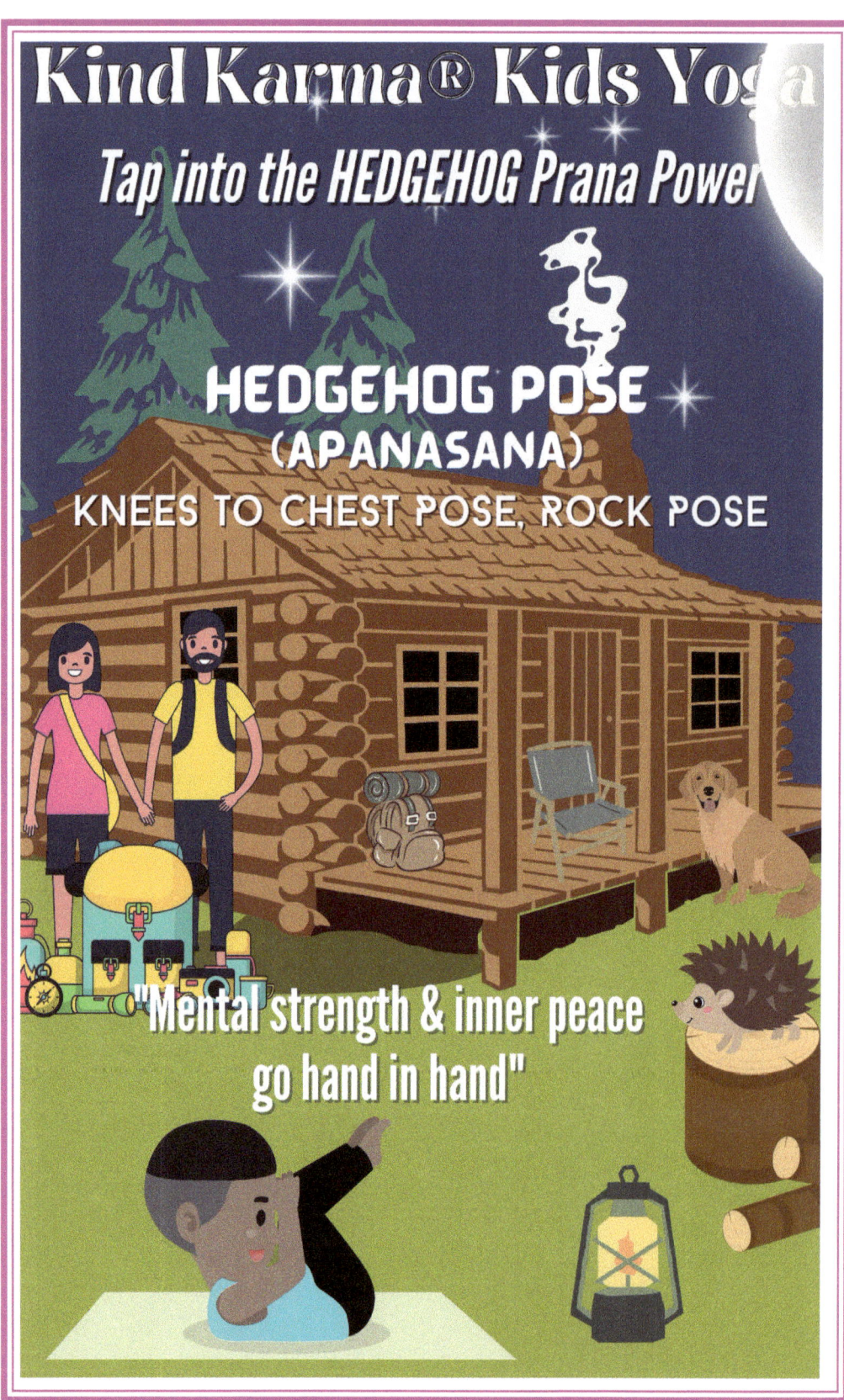

Hedgehog Pose

1. Begin by lying on your back with your legs and arms extended.

2. As you exhale, bring both knees into your chest.

3. Clasp your hands around your shins, slightly below your knees.

4. Gently hug your knees into your chest.

    - Tip: If hugging both knees into your chest is uncomfortable, then hug only one leg at a time.
    - Tip: To keep the back of your neck long, slightly tuck your chin.
    - Tip: Relax your face, jaw and neck.

5. Remain in Hedgehog Pose for three to five breaths, then lower your legs back to the floor.

Benefits

- Releases tension in the lower back.
- Decompresses the spine.
- Relieves abdominal discomfort.
- Increases core awareness.
- Calms the mind and relaxes the body.

Corresponding Element (to embrace your *inner hedgehog* and to help with creating *inner shaman* concepts for class lesson plans)

- Earth.

Hedgehog Attributes (to embrace your *inner hedgehog* and to help with creating *inner shaman* concepts for class lesson plans)

- Refer to the "Associated Animal Attributes" Table.

Corresponding Crystals for Hedgehog Prana Power

- For Calming and Stress Relief: Amethyst, Angelite, Aquamarine, Black Tourmaline, Blue Lace Agate, Celestite, Howlite, Lepidolite, Morganite, Moss Agate, Rose Quartz, Selenite.

Notes

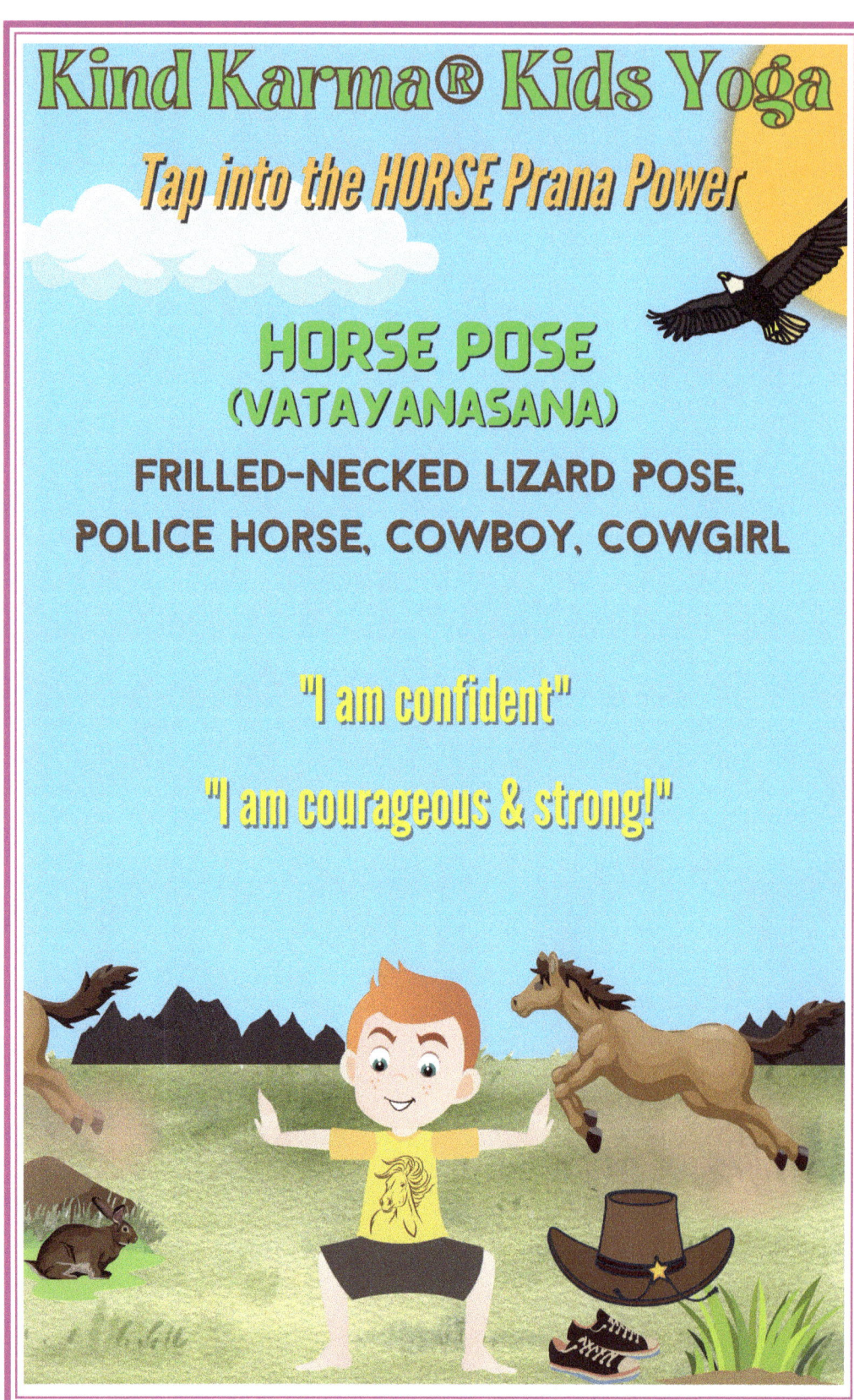

Horse Pose

1. Stand tall in Mountain Pose.

2. Move your feet shoulder-width apart, with your toes slightly pointing outward.

3. As you inhale, reach arms out to the sides, shoulder height.

   - Tip: Slide your shoulder blades downward.

4. Variation: You can press your palms together in front of your chest.

5. As you exhale, bend knees 90 degrees.

   - Tip: Be sure to keep your knees pointed over the feet and your tailbone tucked under your body.

6. Hold Horse Pose for three to five breaths.

7. To end, lower your arms and straighten your knees.

Benefits

- Strengthens the legs, back, shoulders and arms.
- Develops core strength.
- Teaches proper posture.
- Opens hips and thighs.
- Builds physical and mental stamina.

Corresponding Element (to embrace your *inner horse* and to help with creating *inner shaman* concepts for class lesson plans)

- Earth.
- Air (winged horse - mythically, energetically and spiritually).

Horse Attributes (to embrace your *inner horse* and to help with creating *inner shaman* concepts for class lesson plans)

- Refer to the "Associated Animal Attributes" Table.

Corresponding Crystals for Horse Prana Power

- To Increase Confidence and Courage: Amazonite, Aquamarine, Black Tourmaline, Carnelian, Citrine, Dolomite, Garnet, Orange Calcite, Red Jasper, Rose Quartz, Septarian, Spirit Quartz, Sodalite, Sunstone, Tiger's Eye.

Notes

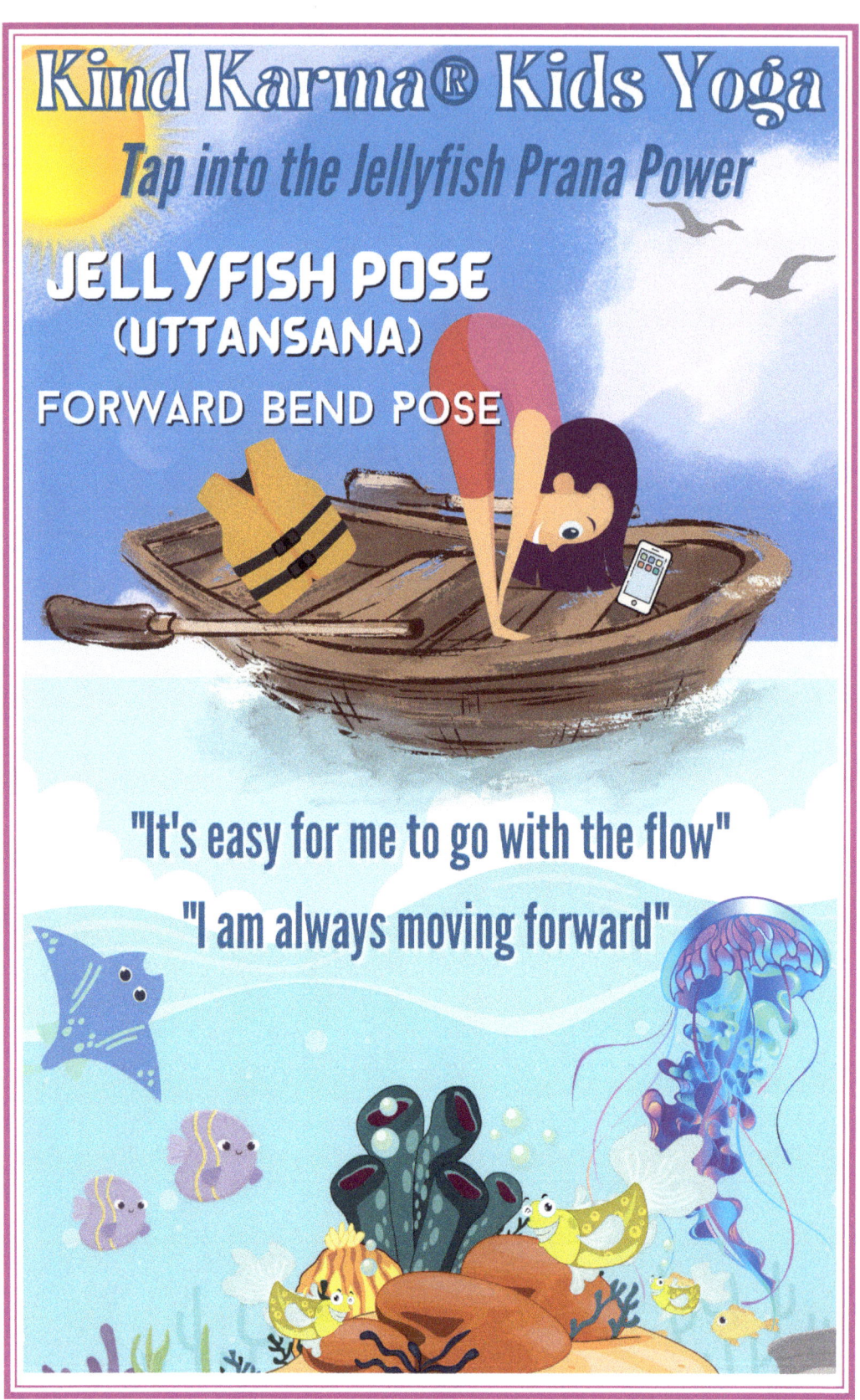

Jellyfish Pose

1. Stand tall with your feet hip-width apart, knees slightly bent, arms by your sides.

2. Inhale, and raise your arms above your head, towards the ceiling or sky.

3. Exhale, and bend forward at the hips, lowering your arms and head toward the floor, while keeping your head, neck and shoulders relaxed.

4. Reach down as far as you comfortably can.
   - Tip: If you cannot reach the floor with your hands, use a yoga block to raise the floor up to you.
   - Variation: you can cross your arms and hold onto the opposite elbows.

5. Hold Jellyfish Pose for three to five breaths.
   - Be sure to relax your face and jaw as you fold forward.

6. To end, bend your knees and slowly roll up into a standing position.

Benefits

- Stretches the neck, back, hamstrings and calves.
- Calms the mind and promotes mental clarity.
- Encourages the feelings of introspection or reflection.

Corresponding Element (to embrace your *inner jellyfish* and to help with creating *inner shaman* concepts for class lesson plans)
- Water.

Jellyfish Attributes (to embrace your *inner jellyfish* and to help with creating *inner shaman* concepts for class lesson plans)
- Refer to the "Associated Animal Attributes" Table.

Corresponding Crystals for Jellyfish Prana Power
- To Promote Creativity: Amethyst, Azurite, Blue Apatite, Blue Lace Agate, Blue Peruvian Opal, Bumblebee Jasper, Carnelian, Citrine, Lapis Lazuli, Moss Agate, Orange Calcite, Rainbow Moonstone, Red Jasper.

Notes

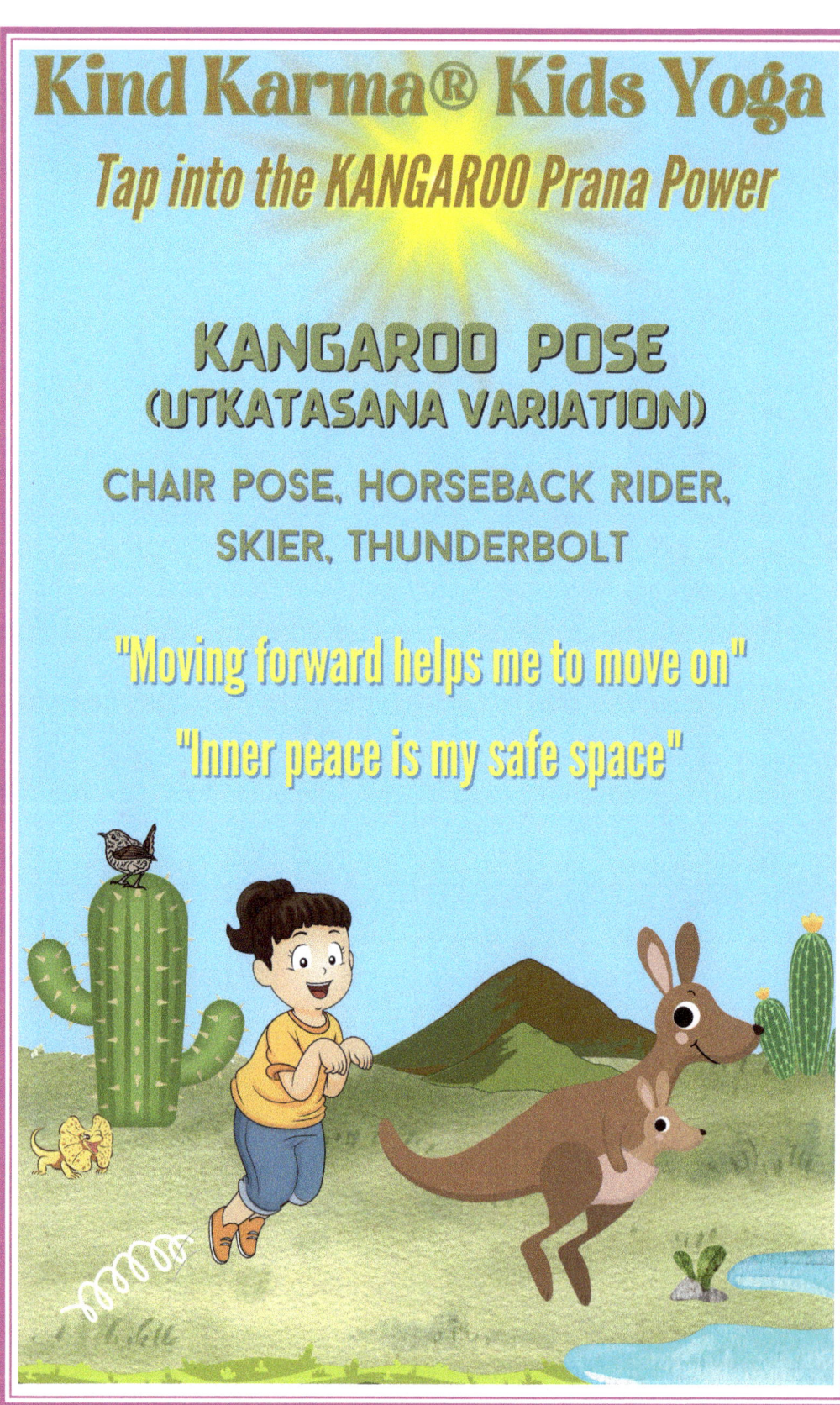

Kangaroo Pose

1. Stand tall with your feet hip-width apart, knees slightly bent.

2. Raise your arms in front of your chest. Bend your elbows and bring your hands together in front of your chest, pointing the fingers down like kangaroo paws.

3. Lower yourself down as if you are sitting on an invisible chair.

4. Now, imagine you are a kangaroo.

5. Hop, bounce and jump as long as desired.

Benefits

- Strengthens the legs.
- Releases pent-up energy.
- Increases alertness and invigorates the body.
- Increases circulation and pumps oxygen to the brain.
- Boosts self-esteem.

Corresponding Element (to embrace your *inner kangaroo* and to help with creating *inner shaman* concepts for class lesson plans)

- Earth.

Kangaroo Attributes (to embrace your *inner kangaroo* and to help with creating *inner shaman* concepts for class lesson plans)

- Refer to the "Associated Animal Attributes" Table.

Corresponding Crystals for Kangaroo Prana Power

- For Letting Go and Moving Forward: Amazonite, Aquamarine, Blue Kyanite, Blue Lace Agate, Chrysoprase, Citrine, Green Aventurine, Howlite, Rainbow Moonstone, Moss Agate, Smoky Quartz.

Notes

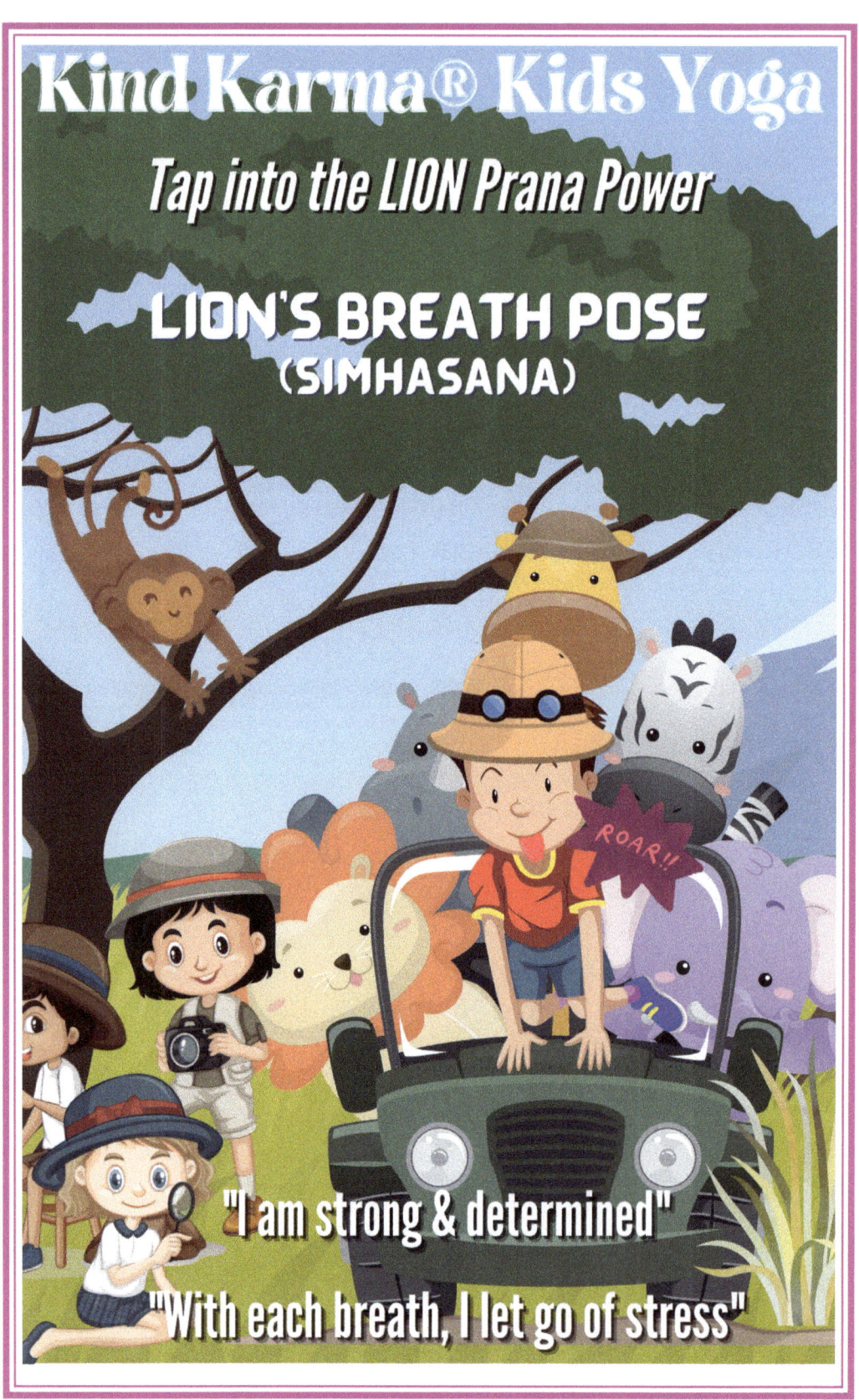

Lion's Breath Pose

1. Begin standing on your knees, then sit back on your heels.

    - Tip: Keep your spine nice and tall.

2. Place your hands onto your knees with your palms resting on the knees. Spread your fingers wide.

3. Take a deep breath through your nose.

4. Next, open your mouth, stretch out your tongue towards your chin, and let your breath out through your mouth and "ROAR" like a lion!

5. Repeat several times.

Benefits

- Releases pent-up energy and reduces stress.
- Increases alertness and invigorates the body.
- Calms the mind.
- Stretches the hips, legs and ankles.

Corresponding Element (to embrace your *inner lion* and to help with creating *inner shaman* concepts for class lesson plans)

- Earth.

Lion Attributes (to embrace your *inner lion* and to help with creating *inner shaman* concepts for class lesson plans)

- Refer to the "Associated Animal Attributes" Table.

Corresponding Crystals for Lion Prana Power

- To Increase Confidence and Courage: Amazonite, Aquamarine, Black Tourmaline, Carnelian, Citrine, Dolomite, Garnet, Orange Calcite, Red Jasper, Rose Quartz, Septarian, Spirit Quartz, Sodalite, Sunstone, Tiger's Eye.

Notes

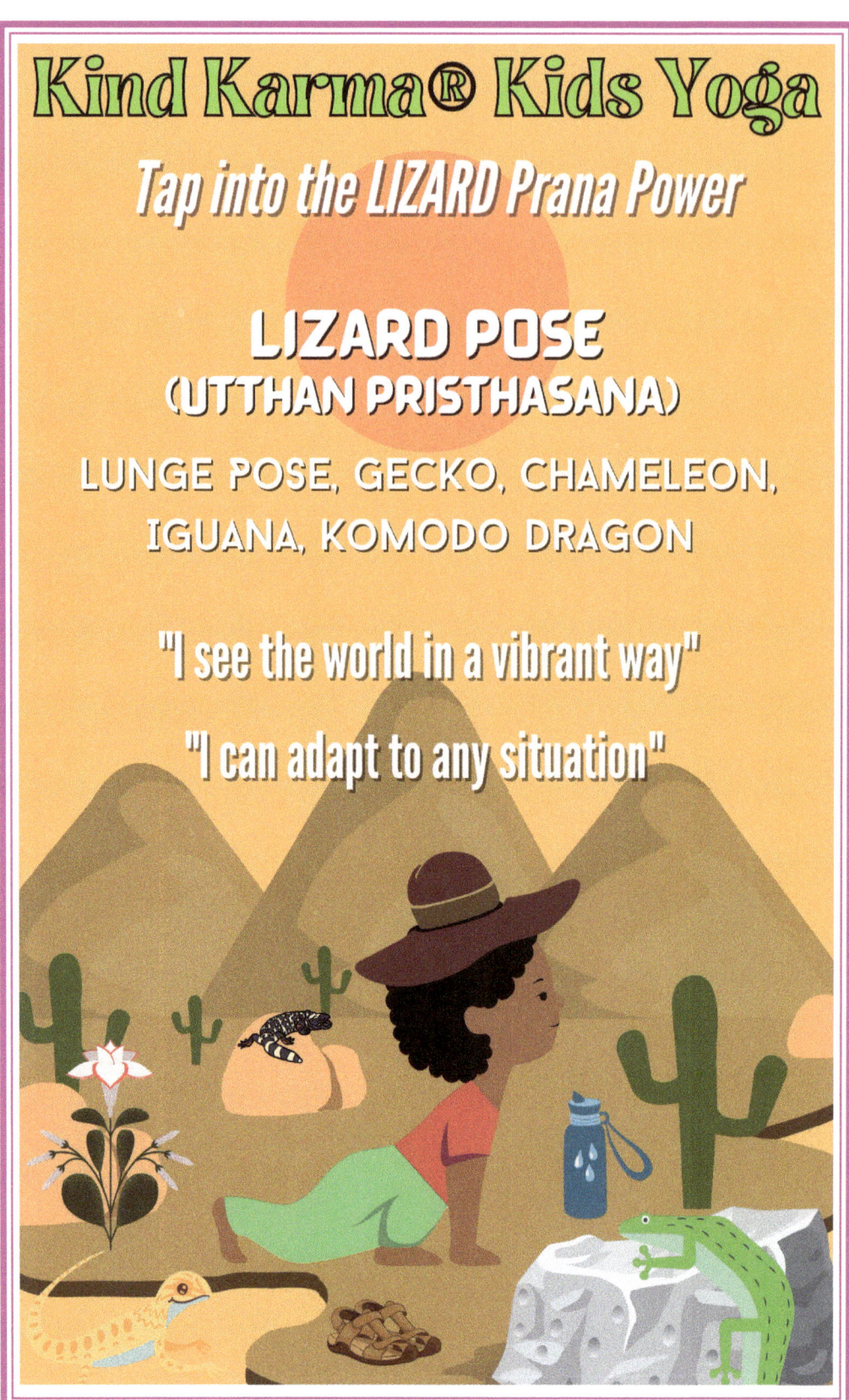

Lizard Pose

1. From Dog Pose (Downward Facing Dog Pose), shift forward to bring your shoulders over your wrists.

2. Gently place your right foot on the outside of your right hand (or, as close as you can), with your right foot facing forward.

3. Stay in this lunge, or Lizard Pose for three to five breaths.

   - Tip: If comfortable to do so, drop your elbows to the ground for a deeper stretch.

4. Option: You can raise the floor by using yoga blocks to rest your hands or elbows.

5. To end, reverse the steps to come out of the pose and go back into Dog Pose.

6. Switch sides and repeat the steps.

Benefits

- Awesome yoga pose to practice after prolonged sitting because it opens the hips, hip flexors and hamstrings.

- Strengthens the inner thigh muscles on the front leg.

- Opens and releases the chest, shoulders and neck.

- Reduces stress.

- Encourages focus.

- Combines the benefits with Dog Pose.

Corresponding Element (to embrace your *inner lizard* and to help with creating *inner shaman* concepts for class lesson plans)

- Earth.

- Fire – some lizards are associated with the fire element.

Lizard Attributes (to embrace your *inner lizard* and to help with creating *inner shaman* concepts for class lesson plans)

- Refer to the "Associated Animal Attributes" Table.

Corresponding Crystals for Lizard Prana Power

- For Adjusting to Change and Adaptation: Amazonite, Amber, Bloodstone, Chrysocolla, Jet, Labradorite, Malachite, Moonstone, Moss Agate, Rhyolite, Tree Agate, Turquoise, Watermelon Tourmaline.

Notes

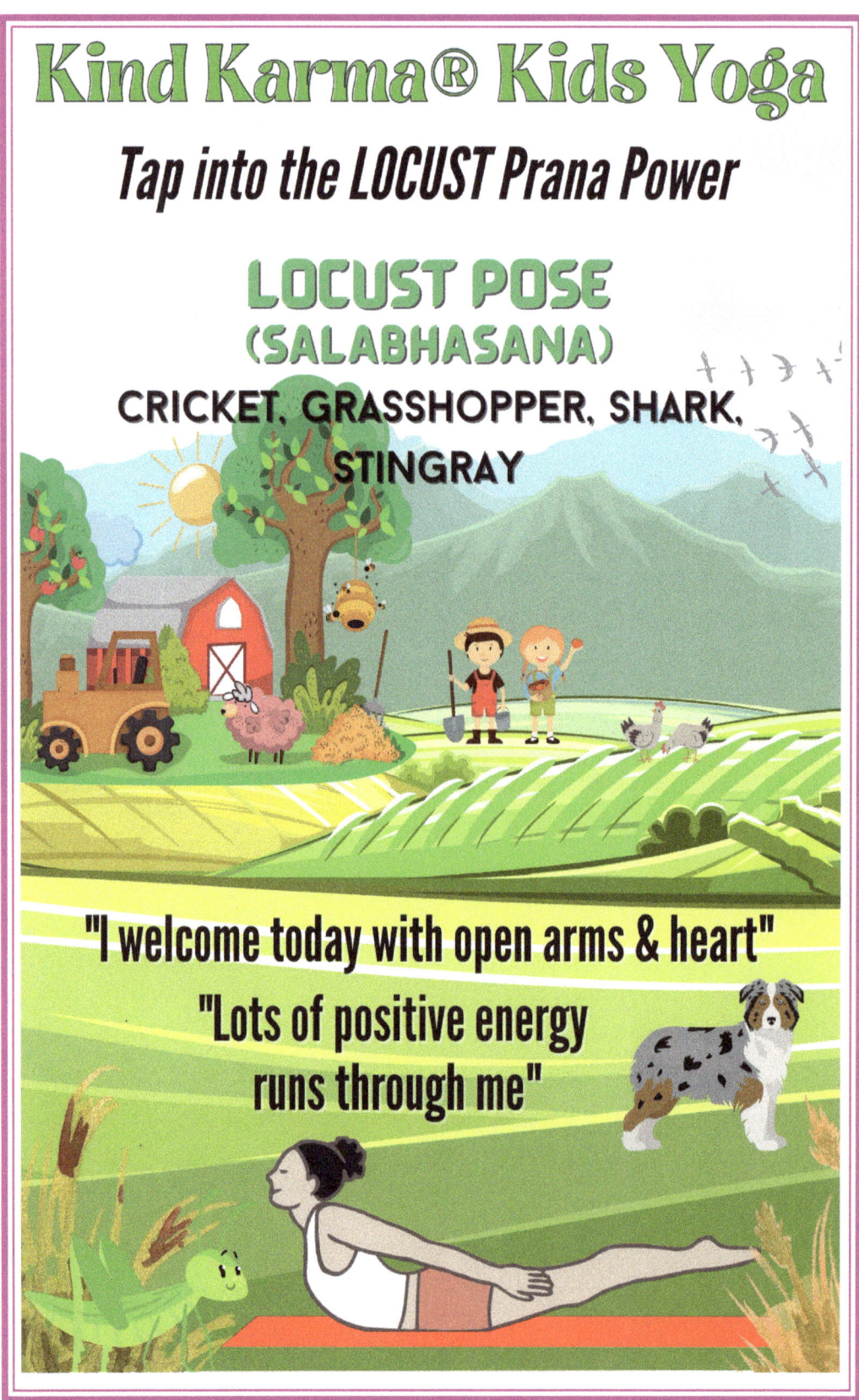

Locust Pose

1. Lie on your belly with your forehead resting on the ground.

2. Place your arms by your sides, palms facing up and finger tips pointing towards your toes.

3. Keeping your core strong and body firm, inhale and lift your head, chest, arms, upper ribs, and legs away from the mat or floor.

    - Tip: Your lower ribs, belly and top of the pelvis should be resting on the mat or floor.

4. Hold Locust Pose for three to five breaths, then lower your entire body to the mat or floor.

Benefits

- Improves posture, opens the chest and counteracts the slouching effects of prolonged sitting.
- Strengthens and tones the back, core, butt and leg muscles.
- Lengthens the spine and improves its mobility.
- Promotes calmness.
- Encourages focus.

Corresponding Element (to embrace your *inner locust* and to help with creating *inner shaman* concepts for class lesson plans)

- Earth - when jumping.
- Air - when flying or launching themselves into flight.

Locust Attributes (to embrace your *inner locust* and to help with creating *inner shaman* concepts for class lesson plans)

- Refer to the "Associated Animal Attributes" Table.

Corresponding Crystals for Locust Prana Power

- For Leap of Faith and Moving Forward: Amazonite, Aquamarine, Blue Lace Agate, Chrysoprase, Citrine, Green Aventurine, Howlite, Mahogany Obsidian, Rainbow Moonstone, Smoky Quartz, Sunstone, Tiger's Eye.

Notes

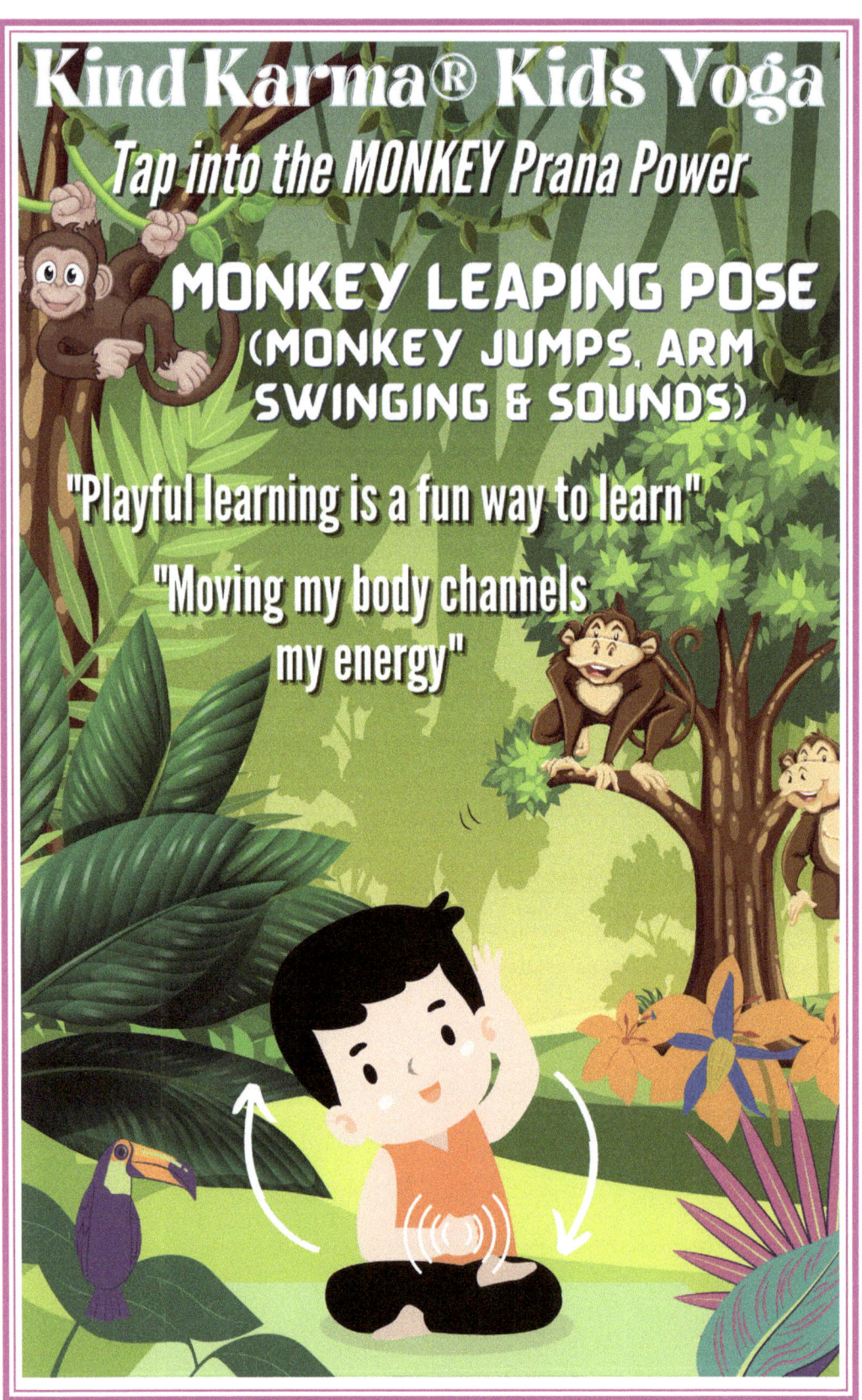

Monkey Leaping Pose

1. From standing, crouch down to a squatting position.

   - Option: You can begin in a seated position instead of standing.

2. Now, from the squatting position, leap up into the air moving your arms up and down like a monkey.

   - Variation: You can make "oooh" sounds as you move your arms.

3. Return back to a crouching or sitting position and repeat several times.

   - Tip: Before you squat again, be sure to stand for a brief moment.

   - Option: You can also tap your belly and chest while you are sitting.

Benefits

- Builds strength: Leaping from squatting to standing and moving your arms up and down will strengthen the leg and arm muscles.

- Strengthens the core muscles.

- Monkey Leaping Pose helps to improve balance skills.

- Jumping, tapping and making sounds helps with channeling energy.

Corresponding Element (to embrace your *inner monkey* and to help with creating *inner shaman* concepts for class lesson plans)

- Earth.
- Fire: With monkeys, energetically, the fire element can arise.

Monkey Attributes (to embrace your *inner monkey* and to help with creating *inner shaman* concepts for class lesson plans)

- Refer to the "Associated Animal Attributes" Table.

Corresponding Crystals for Monkey Prana Power

- To Promote Creativity: Amethyst, Azurite, Blue Apatite, Blue Lace Agate, Blue Peruvian Opal, Bumblebee Jasper, Carnelian, Citrine, Lapis Lazuli, Moss Agate, Orange Calcite, Rainbow Moonstone, Red Jasper.

Notes

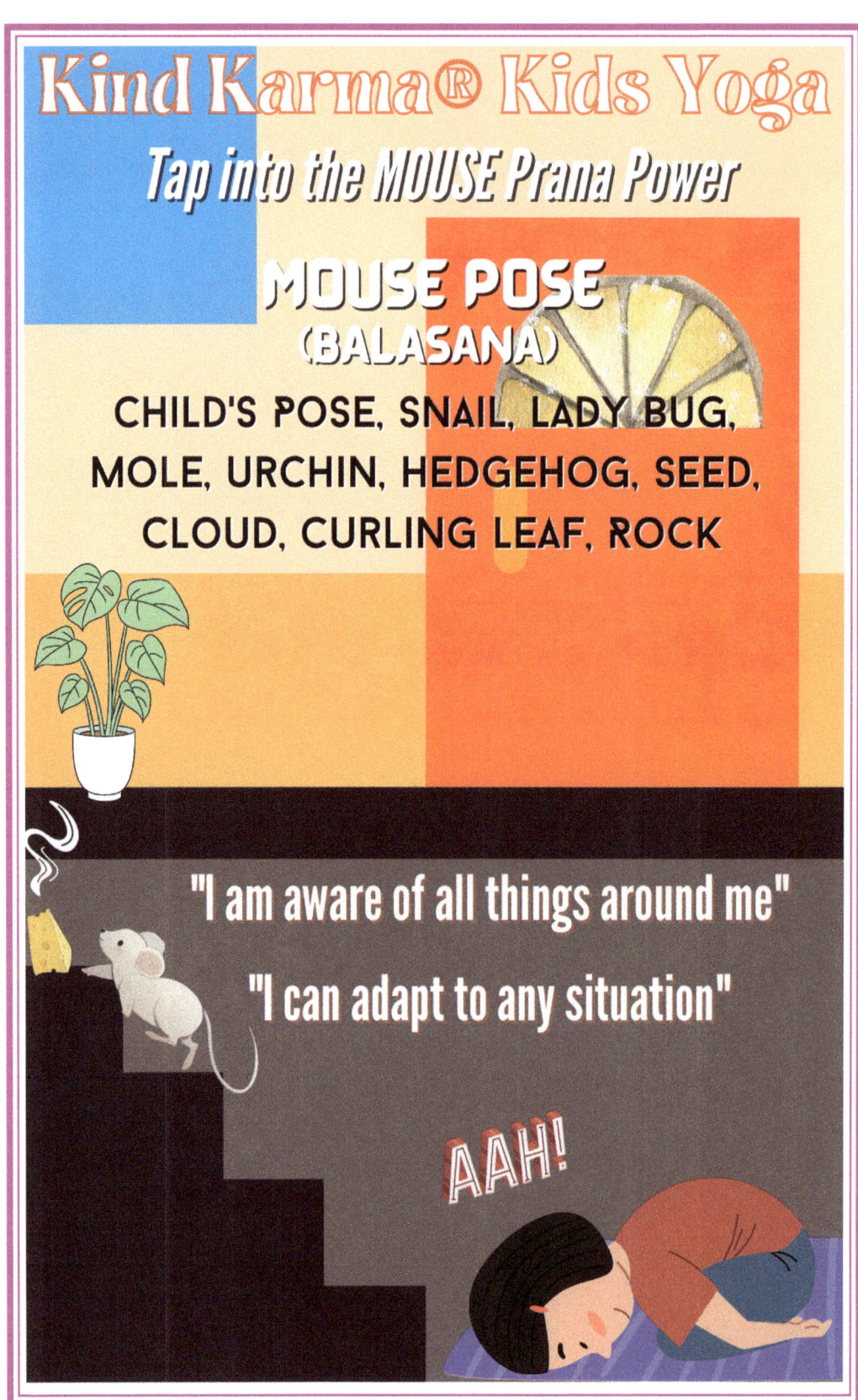

Mouse Pose

1. Kneel on your mat or on the floor, with your big toes touching.

2. Sit back on your heels and separate your knees hip-width apart.

3. Gently lower your head down, and rest it on the floor in front of you.

4. Rest your arms and hands by your sides of your body, palms up.

5. Breathe deeply and relax.

   - Option: Close your eyes.

6. Remain in Mouse Pose as long as desired.

   - Tip: If you experience neck tension, rest your forehead on a yoga block.

Benefits

- Calms the mind, settles the emotions and instills peacefulness.

- Steadies and regulates the breath.

- Decompresses the spine, eases back and neck discomfort, and relaxes the body.

- Stretches the back, legs, knees and ankles.

- Very grounding.

Corresponding Element (to embrace your *inner mouse* and to help with creating *inner shaman* concepts for class lesson plans)

- Earth.

Mouse Attributes (to embrace your *inner mouse* and to help with creating *inner shaman* concepts for class lesson plans)

- Refer to the "Associated Animal Attributes" Table.

Corresponding Crystals for Mouse Prana Power

- To Expression and Communication: Amazonite, Aquamarine, Blue Apatite, Blue Quartz, Blue Tiger's Eye, Carmeilan, Chrysocolla, Clear Quartz, Kyanite, Labradorite, Lapis Lazuli, Larimar, Rose Quartz, Sodalite, Tiger Jasper.

Notes

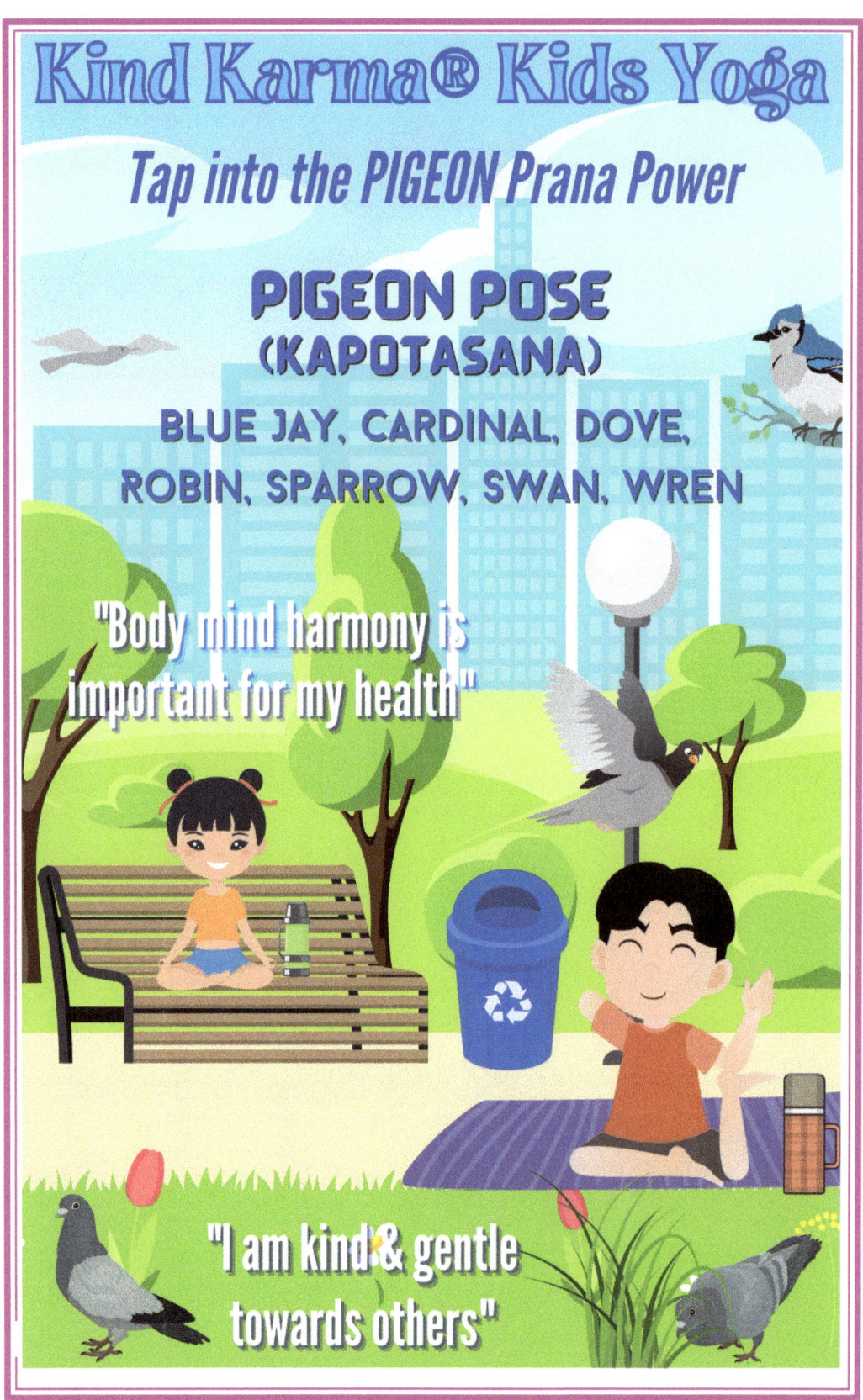

Pigeon Pose

1. Begin in Dog Pose (Downward Facing Dog Pose).

2. Step one foot forward, into a low lunge, placing your foot closer to your opposite hand.

3. Lower your back knee onto the mat or floor, as you tip your front knee to open your front hip.

4. Keep your hands on the floor, and sit up real tall.
   - Tip: Always keep your hips facing forward.
   - Tip: Press your hands into the floor to open your chest and to lengthen your spine.

5. Hold Pigeon Pose for three to five breaths.

6. To end, step your front leg back into Dog Pose, then repeat on the other side.

Benefits

- Stretches the lower back, hips and legs.
- Creates space within the body for deep breathing.
- Releases tension, calms the mind and promotes inner peace.
- Teaches patience.
- Combines the benefits with Dog Pose.

Corresponding Element (to embrace your *inner pigeon* and to help with creating *inner shaman* concepts for class lesson plans)

- Air.

Pigeon Attributes (to embrace your *inner pigeon* and to help with creating *inner shaman* concepts for class lesson plans)

- Refer to the "Associated Animal Attributes" Table.

Corresponding Crystals for Pigeon Prana Power

- For Inner Peace: Amethyst, Angelite, Aquamarine, Blue Lace Agate, Bumblebee Jasper, Celestite, Howlite, Larimar, Lepidolite, Moonstone, Moss Agate, Pink Calcite, Rose Quartz, Selenite, Sunstone, Tree Agate.

Notes

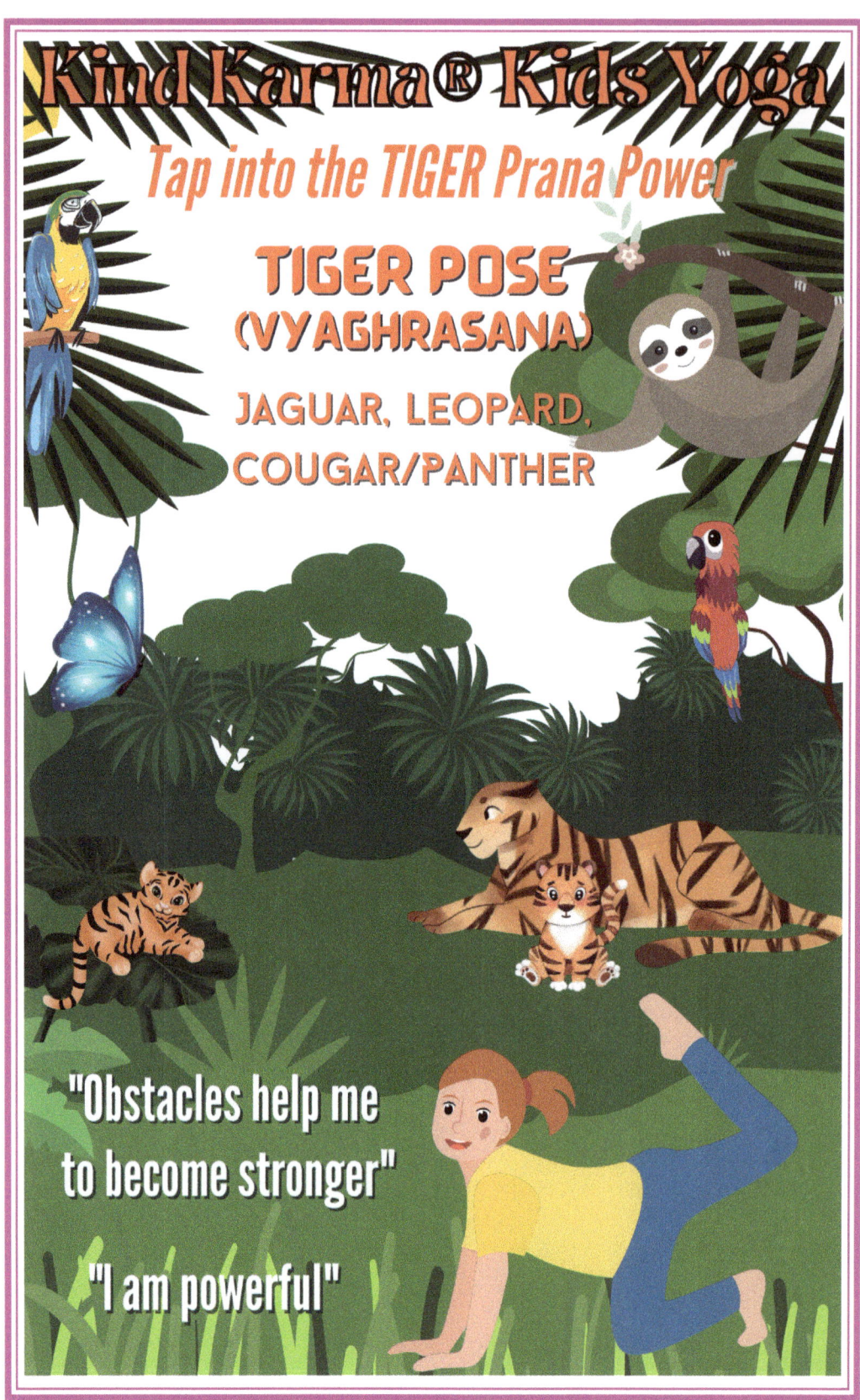

Tiger Pose

1. Begin on all fours. Inhale deeply.

2. Exhale and reach your right foot up towards the ceiling and close to the back of your head. Arch your spine and look up at the ceiling as you bring the foot up.

3. Inhale as you bring your right knee to the forehead, rounding the spine.

4. Exhale again and reach your right foot up back up towards the ceiling and close to the back of your head.

5. Repeat steps 2-4 up to three to five times.

    - Variation 1: You can hold the right foot up for 3 to 5 seconds.

    - Variation 2: When you exhale make a powerful "Haaa" sound out of your mouth.

6. To end, lower the knee back down to the mat or floor, and repeat on the other side.

Benefits

- Warms, stretches and loosens the back muscles and spine.

- Strengthens the back, arms, legs and core muscles.

- Using the "Haaa" sound helps to relieve stress and reduce anxiousness.

- Stretches and opens the hips.

- Promotes body control.

Corresponding Element (to embrace your *inner tiger* and to help with creating *inner shaman* concepts for class lesson plans)

- Fire (energetic nature).
- Earth.

Tiger Attributes (to embrace your *inner tiger* and to help with creating *inner shaman* concepts for class lesson plans)

- Refer to the "Associated Animal Attributes" Table.

Corresponding Crystals for Tiger Prana Power

- To Increase Confidence and Courage: Amazonite, Aquamarine, Black Tourmaline, Carnelian, Citrine, Dolomite, Garnet, Orange Calcite, Red Jasper, Rose Quartz, Septarian, Spirit Quartz, Sodalite, Sunstone, Tiger's Eye.

Notes

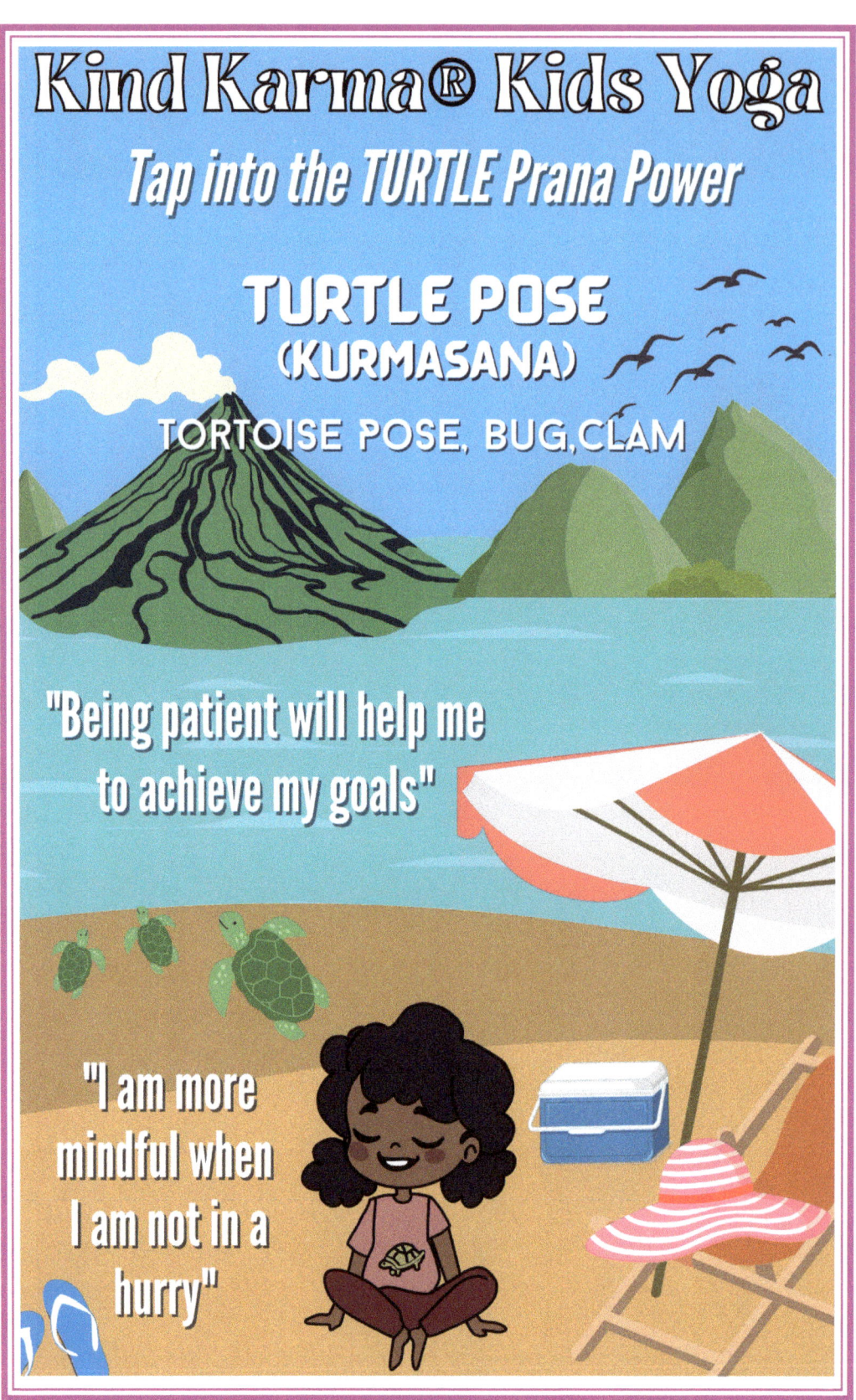

Turtle Pose

1. Begin sitting with your legs straight out in front of you.

2. Bend your knees into your chest with both feet flat on the floor.

3. Slide your feet closer to your body or chest.

4. Next, let your knees fall open to the sides, and slide your hands under your ankles. Lean forward and round your spine creating a shape of a turtle shell.

    - Option: Place your hands where they are most comfortable.

5. Hold Turtle Pose for three to five breaths.

    - Option: You can open the legs wide open.

6. To end, slowly straighten your spine, bring your knees back together, and then straighten your legs back out in front of you.

Benefits

- Stretches the back, neck, arms, legs and inner thighs.
- Reduces stress and calms the mind.
- Reduces back tension.
- Draw your attention and focus inward.

Corresponding Element (to embrace your *inner turtle* and to help with creating *inner shaman* concepts for class lesson plans)

- Water.
- Earth.

Turtle Attributes (to embrace your *inner turtle* and to help with creating *inner shaman* concepts for class lesson plans)

- Refer to the "Associated Animal Attributes" Table.

Corresponding Crystals for Turtle Prana Power

- To Increase Self-Control and Patience: Amber, Aventurine, Black Tourmaline, Blue Lace Agate, Chrysoprase, Dumortierite, Emerald, Green Jade, Howlite, Lepidolite, Septarian.

Notes

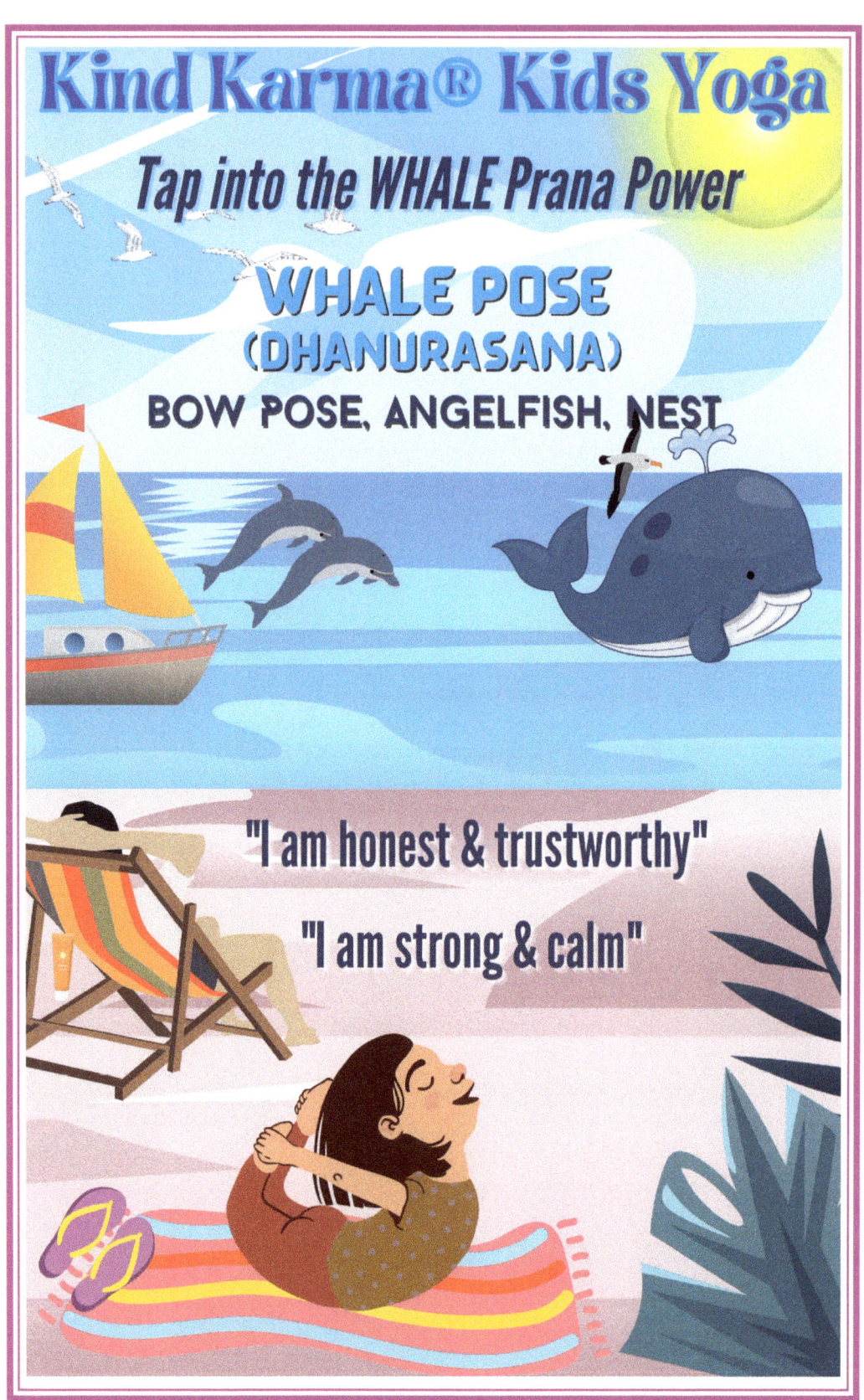

Whale Pose

1. Lie flat on your belly.

2. Bend your knees and reach your hands back with your palms facing each other and the thumbs pointing downward.

3. Try to reach and grasp your ankles or tops of the feet.

4. While holding on to your ankles or feet, press your shins away from you while drawing your feet upward towards the sky.

   - Tip: Pull your belly in and up and navel towards the spine.

   - Variation: If it's uncomfortable to hold onto your ankles then reach as far as you can with your legs still bent and lifted.

5. Now, lift your chest, shoulders, thighs and knees away from the floor. Be sure to keep your head in alignment with the spine.

   - Tip: Keep your thighs, knees and ankles hip-width apart.

   - Tip: Keep your face, jaw and neck relaxed.

6. Remain in Whale Pose for three to five breaths, and then release and lower your legs back down to the floor.

   - Safety Precaution: Always move gently into a backbend.

Benefits

- Stretches the chest, shoulders, arms, belly and legs.
- Improves posture and counteracts the effects of sitting.
- Opens the chest and increases spine flexibility.
- Energizes and invigorates the body.
- Heart opening.
- Builds confidence and self-empowering.

Corresponding Element (to embrace your *inner whale* and to help with creating *inner shaman* concepts for class lesson plans)

- Water.

Whale Attributes (to embrace your *inner whale* and to help with creating *inner shaman* concepts for class lesson plans)

- Refer to the "Associated Animal Attributes" Table.

Corresponding Crystals for Whale Prana Power

- For Inner Peace: Amethyst, Angelite, Aquamarine, Blue Lace Agate, Bumblebee Jasper, Celestite, Howlite, Larimar, Lepidolite, Moonstone, Moss Agate, Pink Calcite, Rose Quartz, Selenite, Sunstone, Tree Agate.

Notes

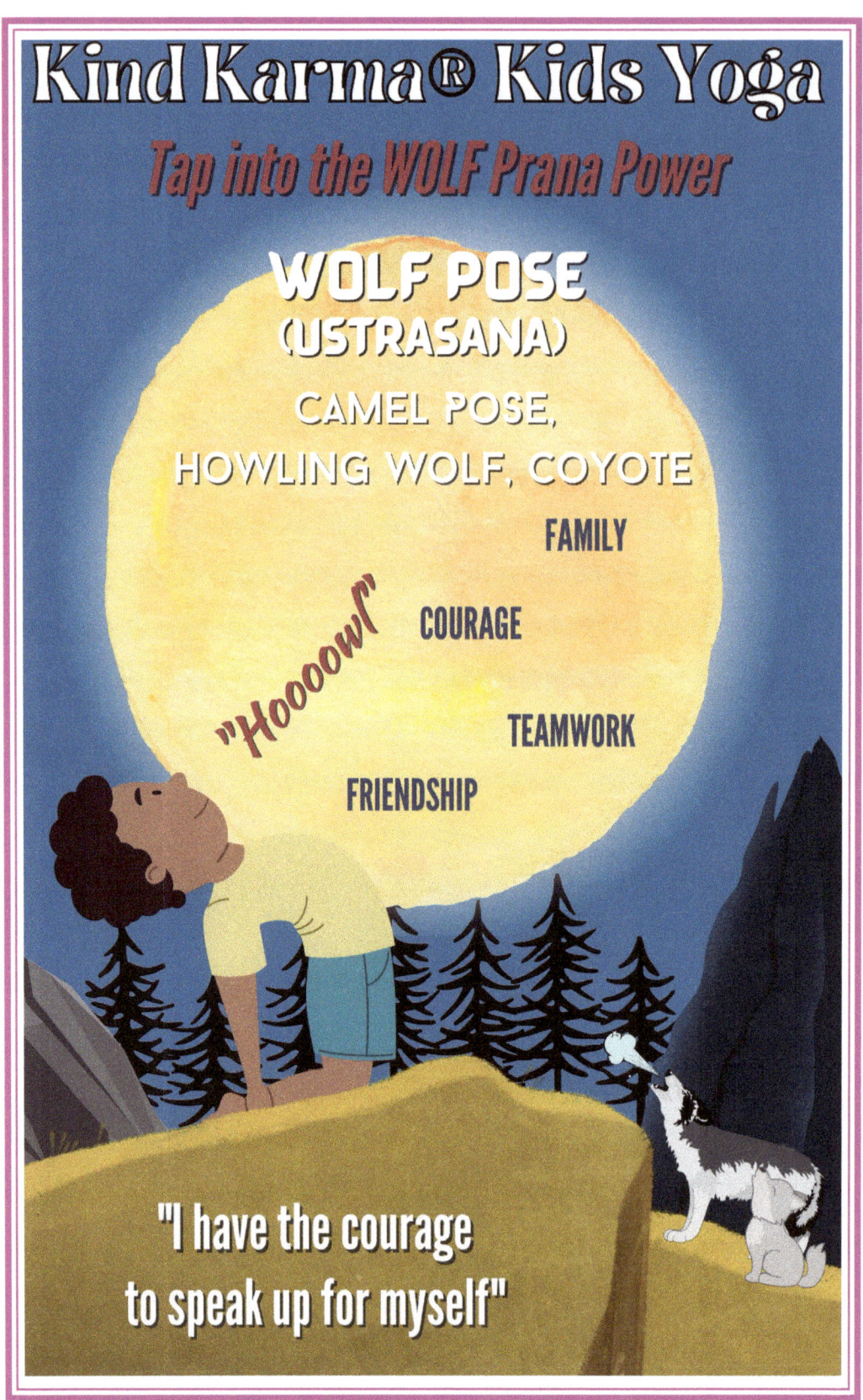

Wolf Pose

1. Begin by standing on your knees hip-width apart, and tops of your feet resting on the floor or mat.

   - Tip: Be sure the knees are no wider than hip-width apart.

2. Place your hands on your lower back, with your fingers pointed down.

3. Lean back until your hands touch your feet. As you move backward, draw your elbows back and pull your navel in and up. This will open and lift your chest and increase thoracic mobility.

   - Safety Precaution: Always move gently into a backbend.

   - Tip: Point the tailbone toward the floor *before* leaning back.

   - Tip: If you are having trouble reaching your feet, use blocks placed on the outside of each ankle or keep your hands on your hips with your thumbs on your sacrum.

4. If comfortable, allow the head and neck to extend backward.

   - Tip: Gaze at the tip of your nose.

5. Hold Wolf Pose for three to five breaths.

6. To come out of the pose, bring your chin to your chest and your hands onto your hips, and slowly come back up to your knees.

   - Tip: Pull in your belly and use your hands to support your lower back.

Benefits
- Stretches the entire front of the body.
- Opens the chest and increases spine flexibility.
- Strengthens the back body including the hamstrings and glutes.
- Improves posture and counteracts the effects of sitting.
- Heart opening.
- Energizing and invigorates the body.
- Builds confidence and self-empowering.

Corresponding Element (to embrace your *inner wolf* and to help with creating *inner shaman* concepts for class lesson plans)
- Earth.

Wolf Attributes (to embrace your *inner wolf* and to help with creating *inner shaman* concepts for class lesson plans)
- Refer to the "Associated Animal Attributes" Table.

Corresponding Crystals for Wolf Prana Power
- For Self-Protection: Amethyst, Aquamarine, Black Obsidian, Black Tourmaline, Citrine, Clear Quartz, Hematite, Pyrite, Fire Agate, Lapis Lazuli, Malachite, Moonstone, Onyx, Opal, Rose, Quartz, Ruby, Selenite, Smoky Quartz, Tiger's Eye.

Notes

DURING THE YOGA POSE, EMPHASIZING THE POSITIVE ATTRIBUTES OF EACH ANIMAL WILL HELP CHILDREN TO BETTER CONNECT WITH THEIR OWN NATURE & TAP INTO THE ANIMAL'S PRANA (ENERGY) POWER

YOGA POSE	ASSOCIATED ANIMAL ATTRIBUTES
BEAR	powerful, confident, brave, patient, direct, intelligent, peaceful, understanding, majestic, resourceful, protective, motherly
BLISSFUL OTTER	kind, happy, playful, joyful, curious, lively, cheerful, dynamic, strong will power, self-control, flexible in body, mind & spirit
BUFFALO	strong, powerful, stamina, grounded, steadfast, divine, linked to nature, protective, inner peace, balance, kind, respectful, stability, abundance
BUTTERFLY	transformative, adaptable, inspiring, joyful, present, giving, nurturing, peaceful, creativity, love, optimistic, lightness of being
CAT	curious, mysterious, magical, independent, self-love, playful, spontaneous, ability to land on your feet, enjoys being unique, affectionate
CATERPILLAR	patient, trust, faith, transformative, optimistic about the future, confident good things happen with change, introspective, doesn't give up
COBRA	reserved, deep inner power, transformative, wise, manifestation, spiritual energy, self-healing, growth, release, magical, shrewd, instinctive

CREATED BY DEAN TELANO

YOGA POSE	ASSOCIATED ANIMAL ATTRIBUTES
COW	loving, gentle, calm, steady, friendly, pensive, warm, motherly, nurturing, quiet strength, stable, giving, family & community-oriented
CROCODILE	powerful, confident, brave, fearless, keen, protective, efficient, precise, patient, vigilant, resilient, crafty, fluidity, clarity, aware
CROW	clever, curious, intelligent, diligent, resourceful, creative, healing, magical, uses laughter as an outlet, community-oriented, fearless, adaptable
DEER	swift, graceful, lightness, aware, transformative, determined, noble, majestic, free spirit, gentle, loving, compassion, caring, generous, powerful
DOG	loyal, faithful, loving, brave, devoted, helpful, enthusiastic, protective, keen, strong, insightful, sensitive, communicative, loving, truthful, patient
EAGLE	visionary, intelligent, skillful, adventurous, brave, observant, powerful, confident, leader, truthful, enlightened, decisive, focused, goal-oriented
FISH	ability to navigate through obstacles, confidence in knowing where you are going, movement, luck, emotional, tranquility, balance, regeneration
FLAMINGO	balance, beauty, synchronization, goal-oriented, vibrant, elegance, compassion, love, serenity, community, cooperation, diversity, steadfastness
FROG	transformative, renewal, nourishing, prosperity, good luck, sensitive, peaceful, cleansing, speaks up, embraces change, handles struggles

CREATED BY DEAN TELANO

YOGA POSE	ASSOCIATED ANIMAL ATTRIBUTES
HEDGEHOG	kind, trust, strength, protective, flexible, calm, happy, resourceful, grounded, centered, peaceful, fortitude, curious, patient, self-dependent
HORSE	confident, brave, powerful, stamina, swift, vitality, proud, noble, steadfast, elegance, free, balanced, powerful, perseverance, friendship, cooperative
JELLYFISH	goes with the flow, peaceful, tranquil, luminous, moves forward, faithful, transparency, sensitive, simplicity, creative, intuitive, yielding, integrity
KANGAROO	moves forward, quick, nurturing, balance, brave, powerful, mobility, protective, energy, motivated, stamina, ability to reach great heights, grateful
LION	courage coming from inner power, vocal, might, strength, family-oriented, protection, majesty, energy, leadership, convicted, respect, relentless
LIZARD	intuitive, seeing the world in color & vibrancy, adaptive, quick-witted, sensitive, imaginative, patient, explorer, determined, self-regeneration
LOCUST	leap of faith, prosperity, energy, courage, virtue, fearless, peacefulness, patience, forward moving, forward-thinking, achieving, independence
MONKEY	social, playful, creative, bold, compassionate, confident, agile, energetic, expressive, light-hearted, clever, curious, mobile, family-oriented
MOUSE	resourceful, expressive, agile, balance, energy, grounded, understanding, eye for details, focus, concentration, creative, adaptable, endurance

CREATED BY DEAN TELANO

YOGA POSE	ASSOCIATED ANIMAL ATTRIBUTES
PIGEON	love, peaceful, gentleness, hope, optimistic, kind, harmony, devotion, calm, purity, grace, innocent, forgiveness, communication, freedom
TIGER	valor, powerful, confidence, fearlessness, pride, strength, resolve, willpower, devotion, passion, protective, royalty, intuitive, independence
TURTLE	diligent, careful, longevity, calm, slow breathing, appreciative, patient, wise, prepared, trusting, enduring, peaceful, determined, receptive
WHALE	communicative, peaceful, compassion, wisdom, contemplative, power, strength, brave, self-reliant, gratitude, magnificence, musical, vibrant
WOLF	protective, cooperation, compassion, power, togetherness, teamwork, instinctual, playfulness, family, friendship, intelligent, brave, expressive

CREATED BY DEAN TELANO

Notes

Section III

Kind Karma Kids Yoga Salutations, Root with Salutes and Flows

The Following Practices Awaken The Inner Shaman:

1. Sun Salutations
2. Tree Salutations I & II
3. 4-Element Warrior Flow
4. I-Am-My-Breath Affirmation Warrior Flow
5. The Power of My Inner Shaman
6. Warrior Poses

Sun Salutations
Kind Karma® Yoga & Shamanism

"Kind Karma® Kids Yoga awakens the inner Shaman that is part of our true nature, which is eternal and unblemished."
– Dean Telano, Creator of Kind Karma® Yoga

From Kind Karma's Yoga perspective, the Sun Salutations are a healing yoga practice that reminds us we are solar beings. The sun, after all, is the source of all heat and light energy on earth. As Kind Karma® Yoga practitioners we emphasize viewing the practice as *circular* in nature, as mother earth and all her inhabitants, revolve around the sun; each day that has gone by we have come full circle.

For us Kind Karma® yogis, every Sun Salutation round completed deepens our connection to the sun and remind us to *shine* from our original *light* essence. Consequently, the invigorating practice of the Sun Salutations balances the mind and body, opens our heart, and awakens our spirit to recognize what we commonly share, deepening our human connections with each other.

During our yoga classes, we teach the children that by practicing the Sun Salutations we are paying homage to the sun. We explain that each yoga pose works collectively to create a dance of rhythmic movement that inspires our celebration and gratitude for the sun, and all that it does for us and nature.

CREATED BY DEAN TELANO

Sun Salutations

Awakening the Inner Shaman

The Sun (called Father Sun), with Mother Earth and Grandmother Moon, form a powerful expression of nature. In some ways they function together as a trinity or a power of three. This trinity is said to influence our lives, watching over us, and guiding us into the deeper aspects of where we came from (ancestors), who we are, and what we are becoming. The trinity, if we are open and mindful of their influence, assists us to grow physically, emotionally, mentally, energetically and spiritually. Through the consistent practice of the Sun Salutations, we deepen our connection with this trinity of nature, particularly the Sun, or Father Sun.

Sun Salutations are breath-based sequences that begin and end with Mountain Pose – *Tadasana*. They combine deep breathing aligned with flowing movement that stretch the entire front and back of the body, build strength, clear the mind, enhance focus and create lots of *heat*. As in nature, the sequence is cyclical, making it easy to become mindfully absorbed in the circuit of repeated movements. Truly, the Sun Salutations are a moving meditation.

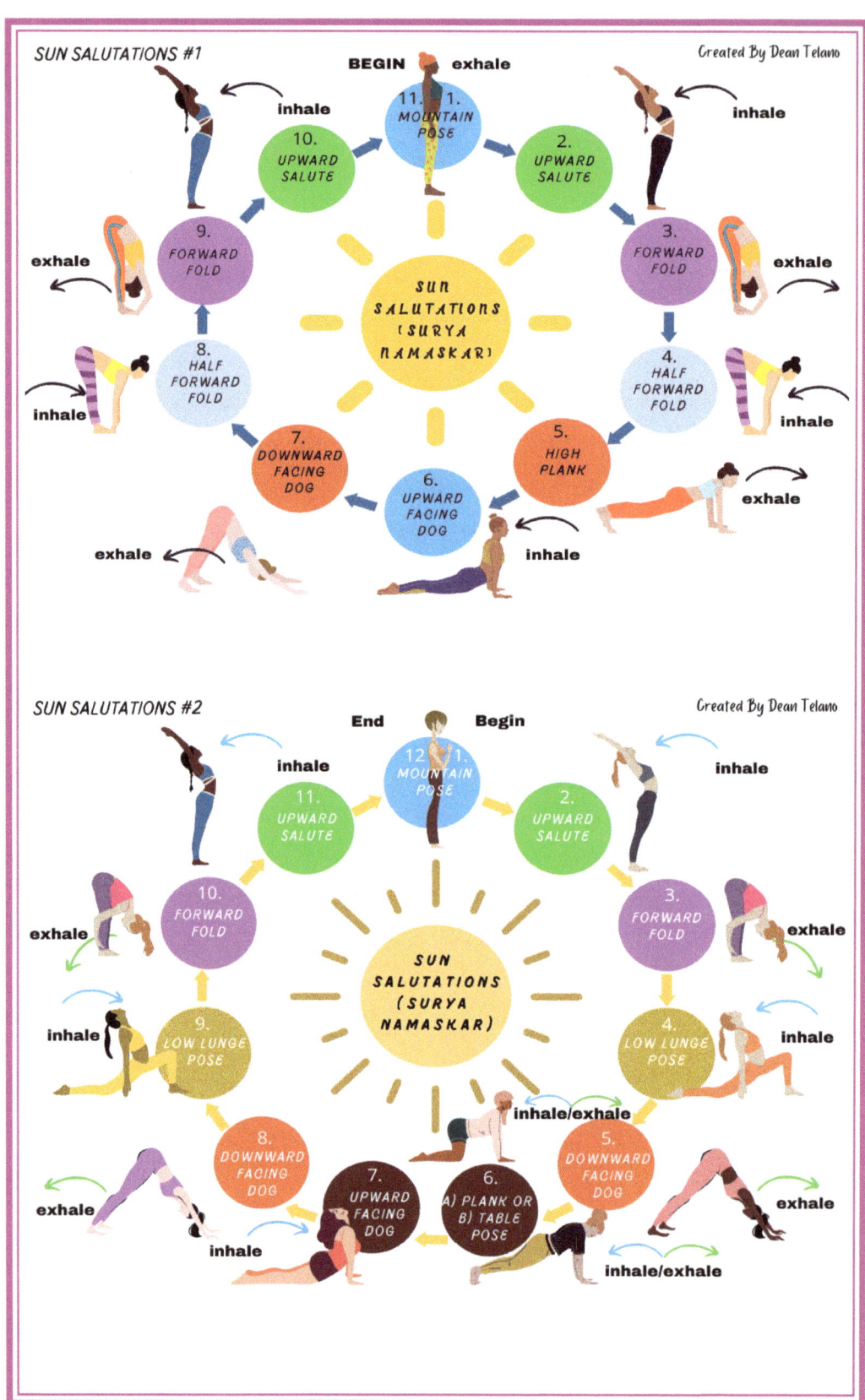

Sun Salutations

Yoga Pose Instructions

1. **Mountain Pose:** Go to Section I: Kind Karma Kids Nature Pose.

    - Place your hands in a prayer *position* by the sternum or chest.

2. **Upward Salute Pose:** Inhale and sweep the arms up above your head into *Urdhva Hastasana*.

    - Reach through the fingertips and lengthen the sides of the waist - side body.

3. **Forward Fold Pose:** Go to Section II: Kind Karma Kids Yoga Animal Poses – *Jellyfish Pose*.

4. **Low Lunge Pose:** Exhale, bend the knees and step the right leg back into a Low Lunge, where the knee rests on the floor or mat.

5. **Downward Facing Dog Pose:** Go to Section II: Kind Karma Kids Yoga Animal Poses – *Dog Pose*.

6. **Plank Pose:** From Downward Facing Dog Pose, move into a high push up position. Your body should be in one straight line, from the crown of your head to your heels.

7. **Upward Facing Dog Pose:** Press the hands into the floor, lift your heart up, arch and lengthen the spine and roll the shoulders down the back.

    - Alternatively, go into Cobra Pose: Go to Section II: Kind Karma Kids Yoga Animal Poses.

8. **Downward Facing Dog Pose:** Go to Section II: Kind Karma Kids Yoga Animal Poses – *Dog Pose.*

9. **Low Lunge Pose:** Exhale, bend the knees and step the left leg forward, as the right knee rests on the floor or mat into a Low Lunge.

10. **Forward Fold Pose:** Step right leg forward into Forward Fold Pose: Go to Section II: Kind Karma Kids Yoga Animal Poses – *Jellyfish Pose.*

11. **Upward Salute Pose:** Inhale and sweep the arms up above your head into *Urdhva Hastasana.*

    - Reach through the fingertips and lengthen the sides of the waist - side body.

12. **Mountain Pose:** Go to Section I: Kind Karma Kids Nature Pose.

    - Place your hands in a prayer position by the sternum or chest.

    - Take a few moments to center and reconnect to your breath before doing the whole sequence on the other side.

Notes

CONNECTING WITH THE TREE SPIRITS

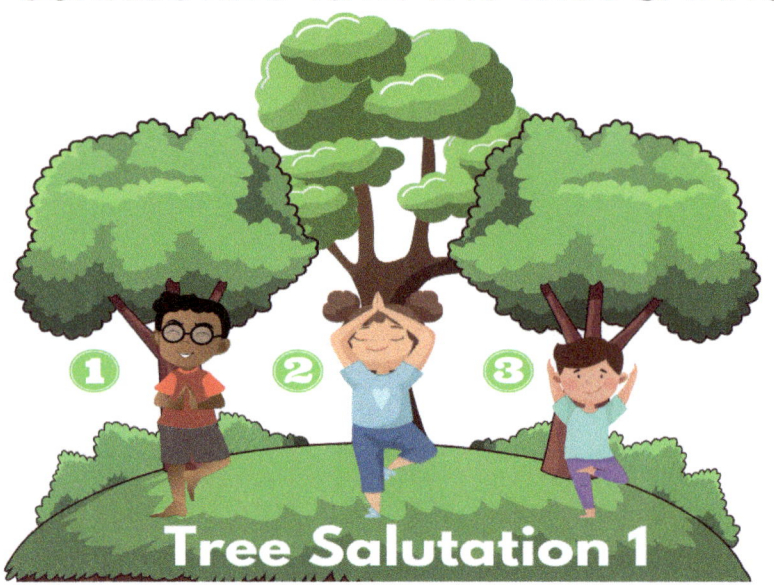

Try to practice each variation of Tree Pose in number progression. Be sure to repeat on the other leg. Practice with your eyes closed, too.

The Shamanic breathwork technique involves breathing in through the nose and out through the mouth in a circular, connected motion.

Nature Interconnectedness Lesson

Practice Tree Breathing: Sit or stand by a tree or trees and breathe in the oxygen that each tree produces. Know when you breathe out carbon dioxide is released, and this helps the tree produce more oxygen. So, trees provide oxygen for each of us and we provide trees with carbon dioxide, which they need. A beautiful relationship!

Don't forget to thank or hug the tree!

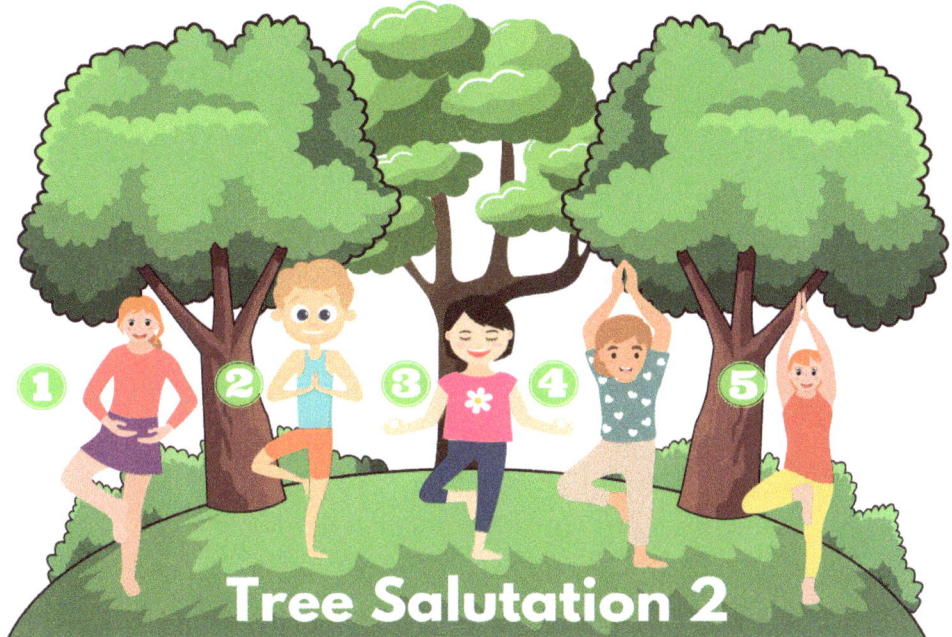

Try to practice each variation of Tree Pose in number progression. Be sure to repeat on the other leg. Practice with your eyes closed, too.

The Shamanic breathwork technique involves breathing in through the nose and out through the mouth in a circular, connected motion.

Nature Interconnectedness Lesson

Practice Tree Breathing: Sit or stand by a tree or trees and breathe in the oxygen that each tree produces. Know when you breathe out carbon dioxide is released, and this helps the tree produce more oxygen. So, trees provide oxygen for each of us and we provide trees with carbon dioxide, which they need. A beautiful relationship!

Don't forget to thank or hug the tree!

Awaken Your Inner Shaman Practice

Illustration 1

"4-Element Warrior Flow"

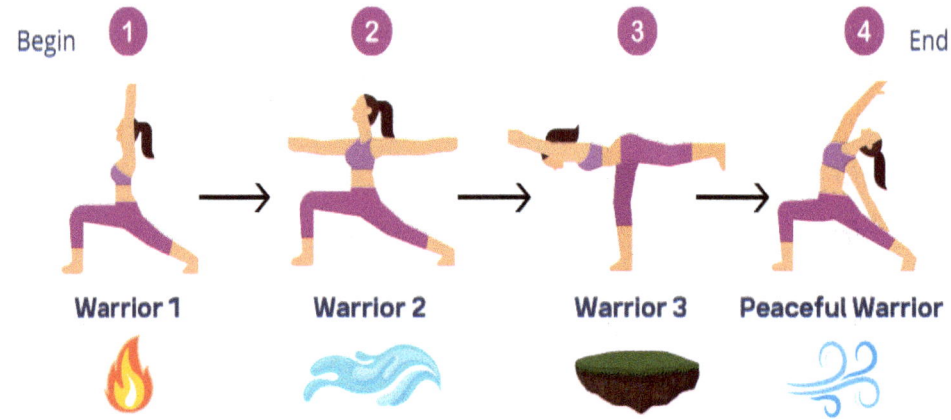

Begin → 1 Warrior 1 🔥 → 2 Warrior 2 🌊 → 3 Warrior 3 🪨 → 4 Peaceful Warrior 💨 End

A Yoga & Ayurveda Perspective: The four elements - earth, water, fire and air, are part of the core of the Kind Karma Kids Yoga Inner Shaman Practice. The four elements represent ideas fundamental to nature and matter. Together, they are a collection of qualities that form the building blocks of who you are, including the physical, mental, emotional and energetic bodies.

Try to hold each warrior pose for 3 breaths as you focus, visualize & connect with each element.

I-Am-My-Breath Affirmation Warrior Flow

The Divine Breath is Within All of Us

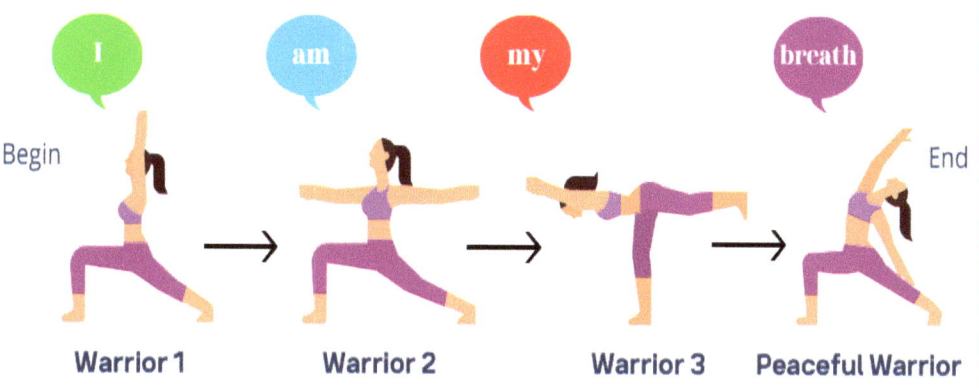

Goal: Breathe in through the nose, out through the mouth.
- Mentally or verbally recite each word of the affirmation as you move into each warrior pose.
- To work on the exhale, and to remain in each pose longer, try to stretch out each word as you say it out loud.
- To change the pace, quicken the recitation and the flow of each pose. Then slow down again.
- Repeat on the other side or leg.

Illustration 2

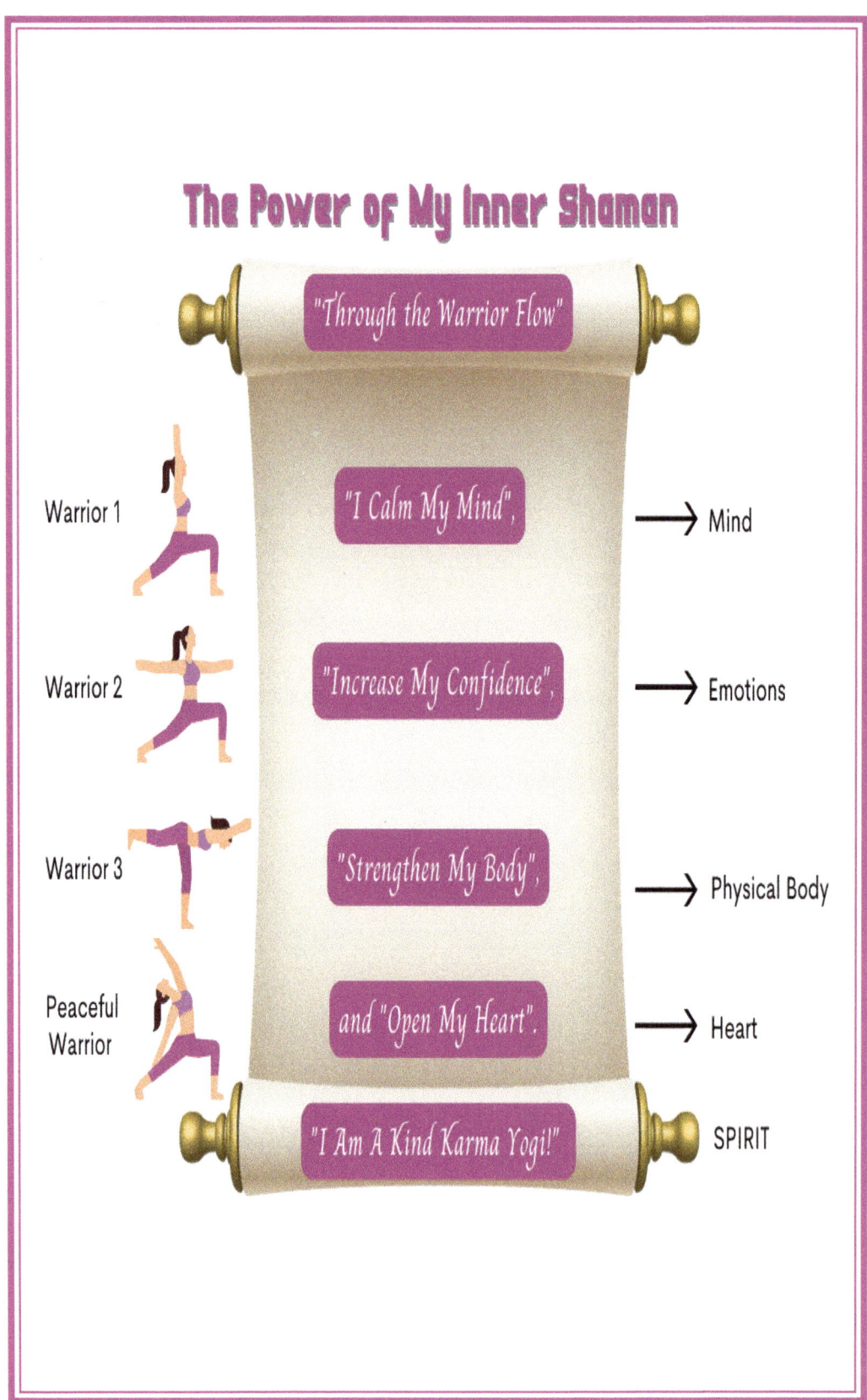

Warrior Poses

Instructions

- Review the *Warrior Flow* illustrations for a visual of each Warrior Pose.
- To learn how to create the *Warrior Pose Flow,* review the prior illustrations.

Warrior I Pose

1. Go to Section II: Kind Karma Kids Yoga Animal Poses – *Deer Pose*.

Warrior II Pose:

1. Begin in Mountain Pose.
   - Go to Section I: Kind Karma Kids Nature Pose.
2. Move your feet so they are wider than hip-width apart.
3. Turn one foot so it's pointing to the side, then bend your knee on the same leg.
4. Stretch your arms out to either side, palms facing down. Try to keep your arms shoulder height.
   - Tip: Look past your extended fingertips.
5. Hold Warrior II Pose for three to five breaths.
6. To end, straighten your front leg, then turn your toes back so they are facing forward again.
7. Switch to your opposite side.

Warrior III Pose:

1. Begin in Mountain Pose.

    - Go to Section I: Kind Karma Kids Nature Pose.

2. Bring your palms together – prayer position – at the center of your chest.

3. Slowly extend one leg back, balancing on the tips of your toes.

4. Hinge from the hips, leaning your torso forward and lift the back leg off the floor. Try to bring your back leg and upper body parallel to the floor as you lean forward.

    - Tip: Extend back through the lifted foot and forward through the top of your head.

    - Tip: Press down through the standing foot, lift the knee and firm the thigh.

    - Variation: Keep palms together or extend arms along ears.

5. Remain in Warrior 3 Pose for three to five breaths.

6. To end, return your lifted leg back to the floor and return Mountain Pose.

7. Repeat on the other side.

Peaceful Warrior Pose (Reverse Warrior Pose)

1. From Warrior III, return your back leg to the floor. Keep your legs wide.
2. Bend at the front knee and keep your body open to the side.
3. Bring your front arm up to the sky, with your palm facing behind you, and lower your back arm down your back leg.
   - Look up at your fingertips of the lifted arm.
4. Hold Peaceful Warrior Pose for three to five breaths.
5. Repeat on your opposite side.

Notes

Section IV

Kind Karma Kids Breathing Exercises (Pranayama) And Meditation Techniques

The Following Practices Awaken The Inner Shaman Through Breathing Exercises And Meditation Techniques That Incorporate:

1. Prana Power
2. Animal & Nature Breathing Exercises List #1
3. Animal & Nature Breathing Exercises List #2
4. Dog Panting Breath
5. Rainbow Breath Moving Meditation
6. 4-Word Finger Meditation
7. Heart Breath Meditation
8. White Light Meditation: 7 Sacred Directions

Prana Power
Benefits of Breathing Exercises for Kids

"Kind Karma Yoga breathing exercises use visualization imagination & sound as gateways to harmonize the body, mind & emotions." – Dean Telano, Creator of Kind Karma Yoga

- Kids love working with the breath!
- It's fun... there's so much fun to be had with breathing exercises.
- Breathing exercises are empowering!
- Increases confidence & enhances self-image & self-esteem.
- Breathing exercises are a valued coping skill, that any child can use any time.
- Self-Regulation: Teaching children breath awareness and breath control encourages relaxation, regulates emotions and provides stress management tools.
- It teaches children how to deal with nerve-wracking, fearful or anxiety-inducing situations.
- Teaches our children to be present and mindful.
- Depending how it's done, it can energize both the body and mind.
- Visualization is a powerful mind-body connection tool.
- Improves respiratory function and strengthens the muscles of respiration, such as the diaphragm.
- Strengthens abdominal muscles.
- Boosts the immune system.
- Improves digestion.
- Clears and eases the mind before school tests or exams, or speaking in front of a class.
- Promotes imagination, creativity and visualization.
- They are wonderful, portable mood elevators.

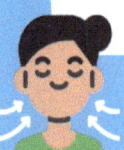 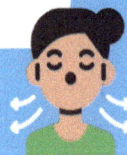

CREATED BY DEAN TELANO

Animal & Nature Breathing Exercises (Pranayamas) to Promote Nature Interconnectedness & Self-Regulation: List #1

BUFFALO BREATHING

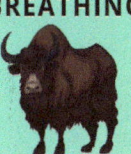

In Buffalo Pose, take in deep inhales through the nose followed by long exhales through mouth. Feel each exhale root out through the feet and into the earth. During every exhale feel grounded, centered and calm. Practice as long as is needed.

EAGLE BREATHING

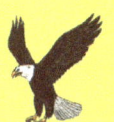

In Eagle Pose, inhale twice through the nose (eagles breath through slits near top of the beak) followed by one long exhale through the mouth. Be sure the exhale is longer than both of the consecutive inhales combined. Clears the mind, relaxes the body.

WOLF BREATHING

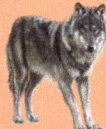

In a gentle Camel Pose (modify if needed), inhale through nose and exhale powerfully, making a long howl. Repeat for 3-5 breaths, then go into Mouse Pose (this is a counter pose for Camel pose). This will release excess energy, stress or tension. The mild inversion (Mouse Pose) will clear the mind.

BEAR BREATHING

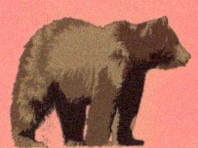

In Bear Pose, take in slow, deep breaths through your nose. After each inhale, hold or pause your breath for a second or two. Release the breath through the mouth. Breath pauses release anxiety and stress, and strengthens the diaphragm. Can be practiced seated or on all fours. As needed.

CROCODILE BREATHING

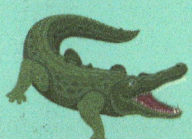

On you belly (prone position) stack your arms underneath your chin and rest your head on your hands, palms facing down. Take in deep, long belly breaths. Floor breathing teaches the child how to breathe using the diaphragm and belly. This breath is calming and soothing. As needed.

CREATED BY DEAN TELANO

Animal & Nature Breathing Exercises (Pranayamas) to Promote Nature Interconnectedness & Self-Regulation: List #2

MONKEY BREATHING

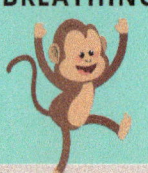

In Monkey Leaping Pose, when jumping up and down tap your chest with your fists. As you tap your chest make the following sounds: *Ooh, Ooh, Ooh, Ah, Ah*. After making the sounds, sit back down and repeat 3-5 times. The jumping, tapping and sounds will channel energy and release anxiety, stress and worry.

LION'S BREATH

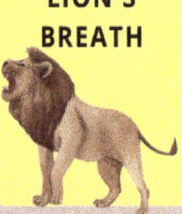

Begin on your knees, then sit back on your heels – Lion Pose. Next, spread your fingers wide, and press your hands onto your knees. Take a deep breath in through your nose. Open your mouth, stretch out your tongue, open your eyes wide, through your mouth release a loud "ROAR!" A *HAAA* sound can be used.

BUMBLE BEE BREATH

Sitting with a nice straight back, gently block your ears with your thumbs and place your index fingers softly on your brow. Your remaining fingers can gently fall across your eyes to close them. Breathe in through your nose with your mouth closed, and then as you breathe out make a long *hummm* sound.

SNAKE BREATH

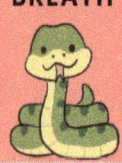

Sitting with a nice straight back, place one palm on your knee and the other on your belly to feel the lungs and diaphragm working as you breathe. Next, slowly breath in through your nose, filling the lungs from the bottom up. Finally, slowly *HISS* (or, *SSS*) out the breath, seeing how long you can exhale.

BUNNY BREATH

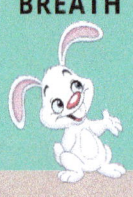

Sit on your knees like a bunny, keeping your back straight and chest lifted. Next, take in three quick sniffs in through your nose. When completed, breathe out through your mouth with a long, smooth *SIGH* or *AAH* sound. Over time, try to increase the number of your inhalations and lengthen your exhalations.

CREATED BY DEAN TELANO

Dog Panting Breath

Mindful Breathing is a Powerful Form of Mindful Meditation Practice

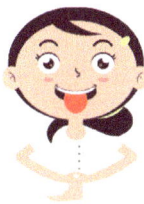
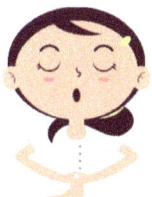
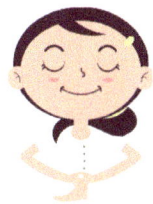

Dog Panting with tongue out

If it's uncomfortable sticking your tongue out, then do *cannon breath*, where your mouth is opened in an 'O' shape & tongue relaxed

Practice Meditation for 2-3 minutes after *dog panting breath*

- Sit Comfortably. Place your hands on your knees or in your lap. Option: You can sit on your heels.
- Open your mouth wide and stick your tongue out all the way. Keep it out as you rapidly breathe in and out through your mouth. Pant like a dog would.
- Pull you belly in towards your spine with every exhale. All your breathing should take place through your mouth. Don't hold back now – pant!
- Continue for 1-2 minutes. If 1 minute is too stressing for beginners, start with 15-20 seconds and gradually reach up to 1 and then up to 2 minutes.
- End with a closed-eye meditation for 2-3 minutes.

RAINBOW BREATH MOVING MEDITATION

*Visualization
 *Imagery

*Moving with the Breath
 *Awareness

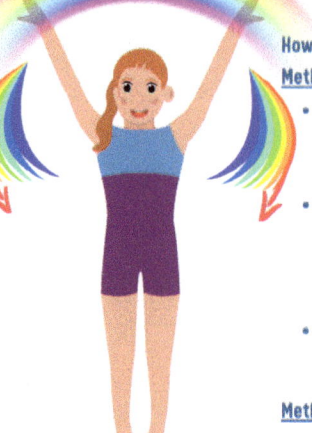

Begin in MOUNTAIN POSE
1. Stand with feet hip distance apart and arms relaxed at your sides, with palms slightly facing outward.
2. Keep your feet parallel to each other. Root your feet.
3. Lengthen your tailbone down as you draw your navel in.
4. Allow your chest to expand as you relax your shoulders down.
5. Keep your chin parallel to floor and gaze forward (or close your eyes).
6. Raise your arms over head & then lower your arms back to your sides.
7. Repeat at least 7 times – for each color of the rainbow (and chakra).

How to do Rainbow Breath Meditation
Method #1: Breath in nose & out mouth.
- Each time you swing your arms upward (from the sides of your body) visualize the colors of each rainbow ray.
- Start by visualizing the red color entering the body as you inhale. As you breath out, lower your arms & visualize the red color leaving the body.
- Repeat with rest of the colors: orange, yellow, green, blue, indigo & violet.

Method #2: Breath in nose & out mouth.
- Have the child decide what color they want to imagine or what color they feel they need to center themselves or to feel good.

*Increases Mindfulness
*Enhances Focus
*It's FUN!

*Reduces stress, nervousness, worry, tension & restlessness

*Channels excess energy
*Helps to mange emotions

4-Word Finger Meditation
"I-Am-My-Breath"

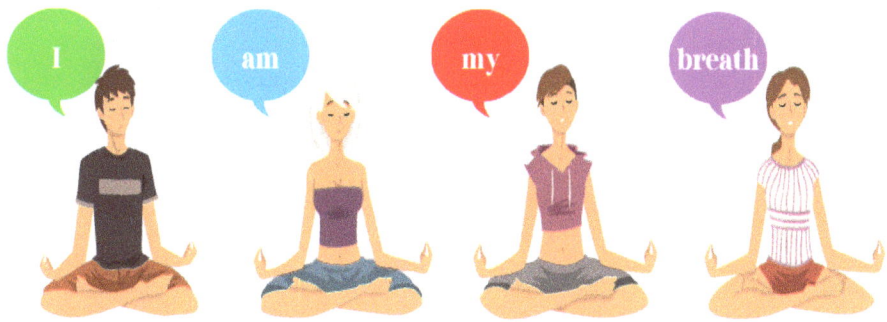

How To Practice I Am My Breath Meditation: Keep Eyes Closed Throughout The Meditation

- Find a comfortable seating position. Cross the legs and keep the spine straight. Rest your hands or wrists on top of your knees, with your palms facing the upward.
- While saying "I", touch your thumbs and index fingers together on both hands.
- While saying "Am", touch your thumbs and middle fingers together on both hands.
- While saying "My", touch your thumbs and ring fingers together on both hands.
- While saying "Breath", touch your thumbs and little fingers together on both hands.
- Repeat for 1-3 minutes. Build to 3-5 minutes.
- To end: Inhale, then exhale. Stretch the spine, with your arms reaching up as far as possible. Spread the fingers wide, taking several deep breaths. Relax.

Awaken Your Inner Shaman
Heart Breath Meditation

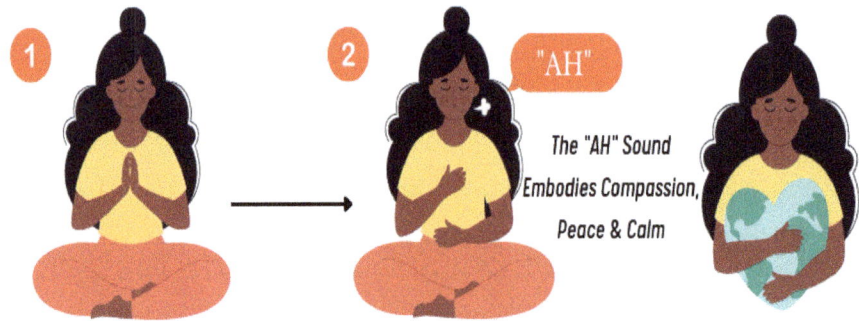

1. Begin with your hands in prayer position. Pray or offer gratitude.
2. Place your hands on your chest & belly. Imagine you have a very BIG heart, growing with each breath.
3. Focus your awareness on your chest and your BIG HEART.
4. Breath in and out through your mouth - like a gentle breeze, filling your entire chest or *Heart Chakra Space*.
5. Now, recite the sound *AAAH* several times, allowing the sound and its vibration to fill your entire chest or *Heart Chakra Space*. Feel how your heart opens and vibrates with the *AAAH* sound.
6. After 2-3 minutes, return to regular breathing & let your hands float down to rest into your lap.

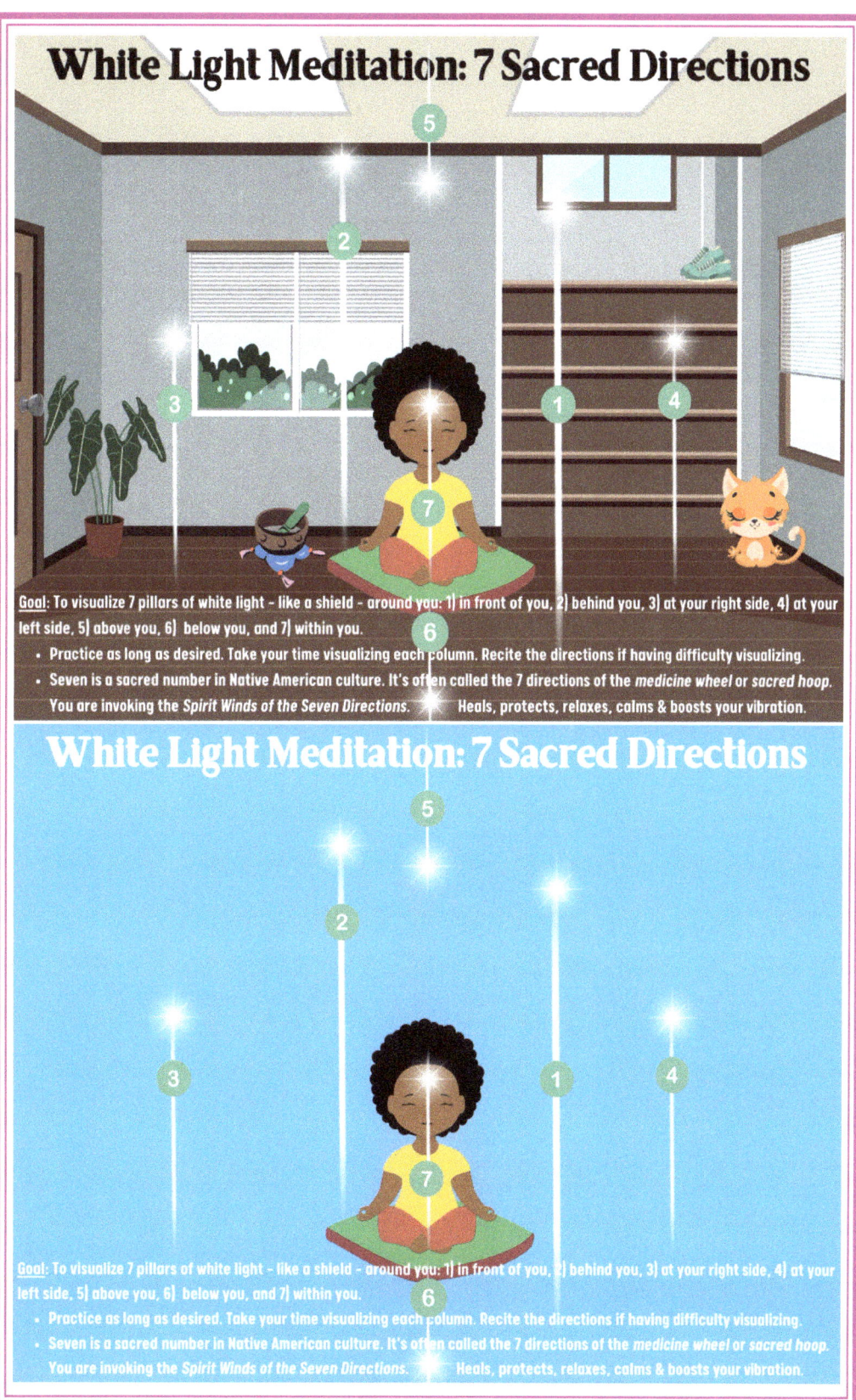

Notes

SECTION V

Kind Karma Kids Yoga: Medicine Wheels, Seven Sacred Directions, Four Elements, Crystals

The Medicine Wheel Or Sacred Hoop, And The Following Illustrations Will Help To Guide You How To Create Ways To Awaken The Inner Shaman During A Kind Karma Kids Yoga Practice.

1. Significance of The Circle Shape & Medicine Wheel
2. Medicine Wheels
3. The Four Elements of Nature's Magic
4. The Four Elements of The Human Body
5. Crystals & The 4 Elements
6. The Seven Sacred Directions of The Medicine Wheel or Sacred Hoop
7. Key Aspects of The Medicine Wheel for Lesson Plans

Significance of the Circle Shape & Medicine Wheel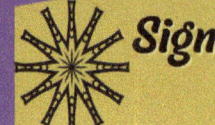

Symbolism of the Circle Shape
(In Kind Karma Yoga, We Call it the Circle of Light & Compassion)

- Represents the Divine Source or Spirit.
- Represents the interconnectivity of all aspects of one's being, including the deep connection we have with the nature.
- Unity, union, inclusion & togetherness.
- Totality, wholeness & completion.
- Perfection & harmony.
- Represents the circle of life, circle of wisdom & circle of self-awareness.
- Represents a spiritual journey.
- Symbolizes focus & centering.
- Symbolizes mobility.
- Symbolizes nurturing.
- Represents evolution as a process of transformation.
- A circle has no beginning and no end. In this sense, a circle represents eternity or infinity.
- All cyclic movements, as in the cyclic nature of the universe.
- Often represents the Sun.
- Cosmic unity, celestial bodies & the infinite nature of energy.
- Creating or visualizing a circle is often used as a form of protection.

The above information can be incorporated into your Kind Karma Kids Yoga class lesson plans or practice

CREATED BY DEAN TELANO

MEDICINE WHEEL #1 - SACRED HOOP
Medicine Wheel Theme

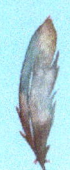

Teaching Idea
In a circle, teach about the medicine wheel using the season, direction, color & elements as you involve the children.

- **North** — Winter, White, Air/Wind
- **West** — Autumn, Black, Earth
- **East** — Spring, Yellow, Fire
- **South** — Summer, Red, Water
- **Center** — SPIRIT or Me

Teaching Idea
In a circle, teach how we are all intrinsically connected with the earth and her cycles, nature and to one another. Togetherness.

Created By Dean Telano

MEDICINE WHEEL #2 - SACRED HOOP
Medicine Wheel Theme

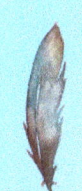

Teaching Idea
Using one or more of the the animals shown on the Medicine Wheel, locate the animal(s) in the book and have the children practice that specific yoga animal pose.

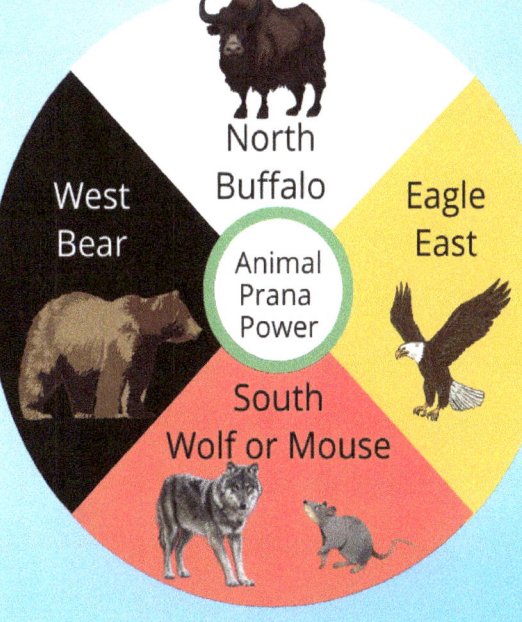

- **North** — Buffalo
- **West** — Bear
- **East** — Eagle
- **South** — Wolf or Mouse
- **Center** — Animal Prana Power

Teaching Idea
Practicing the animal poses, refer to the chart & teach the attributes associated with each of the 4 animals. Have the child feel the *Prana Power* by repeating the specific animal affirmation(s).

Created By Dean Telano

Medicine Wheel #3 - Sacred Hoop
Medicine Wheel Theme

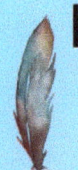

Element: Air/Wind
- 5 Pointed Star Pose
- Half Moon Pose

Element: Earth
- Mountain Pose
- Tree Pose

Nature Poses

Element: Fire
- Sun Salute
- Volcano Pose

Element: Water
- Lotus Pose
- Waterfall Pose

<u>Teaching Idea</u>
Teach the children the "nature" poses that correspond to the particular element. The poses can be found inside the book with their nature affirmations.

<u>Teaching Idea</u>
All ten nature poses in the book can be taught. The two rainbow poses are very special (like all rainbows!) and can be taught with any of the four elements.

Created By Dean Telano

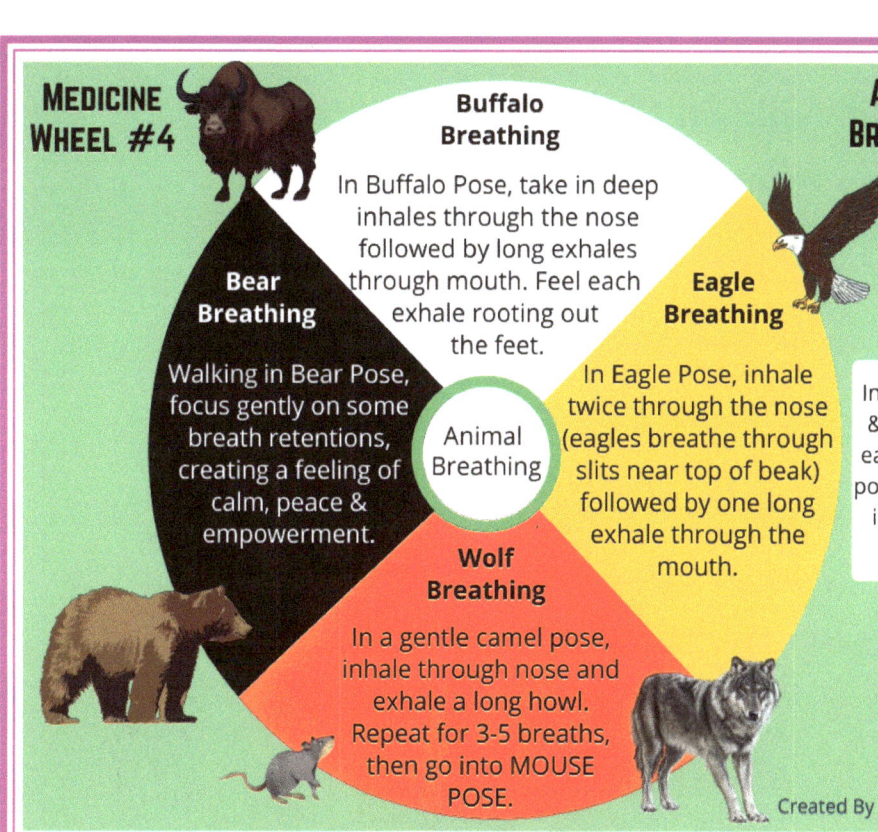

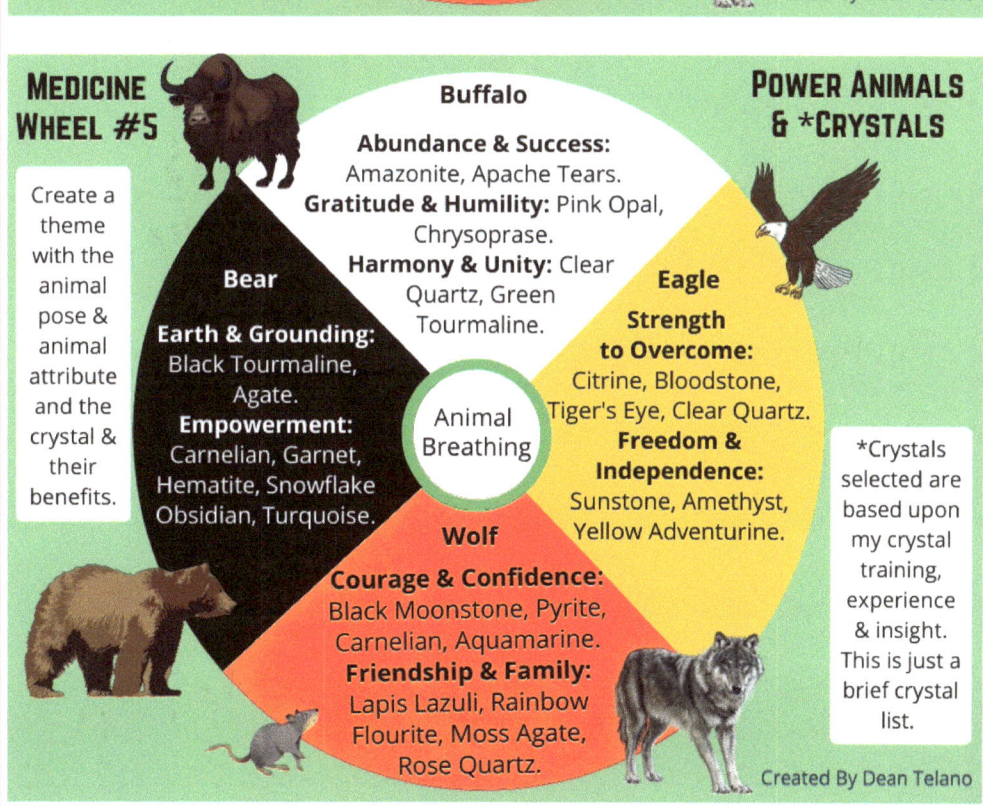

Kind Karma Kids Yoga
The Four Elements of Nature's Magic

The 4 Elements Sustain All Living Beings & Make Life on Earth Possible

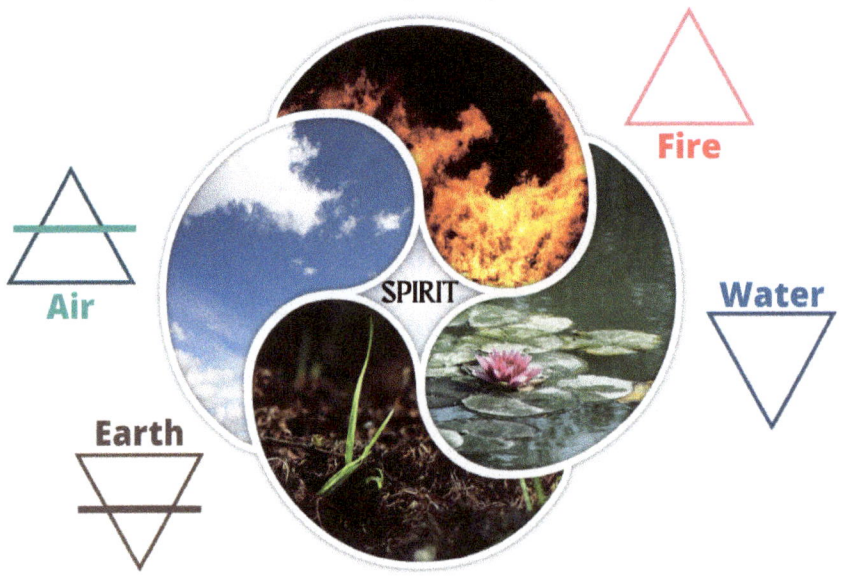

Notes

The Four Elements of the Human Body

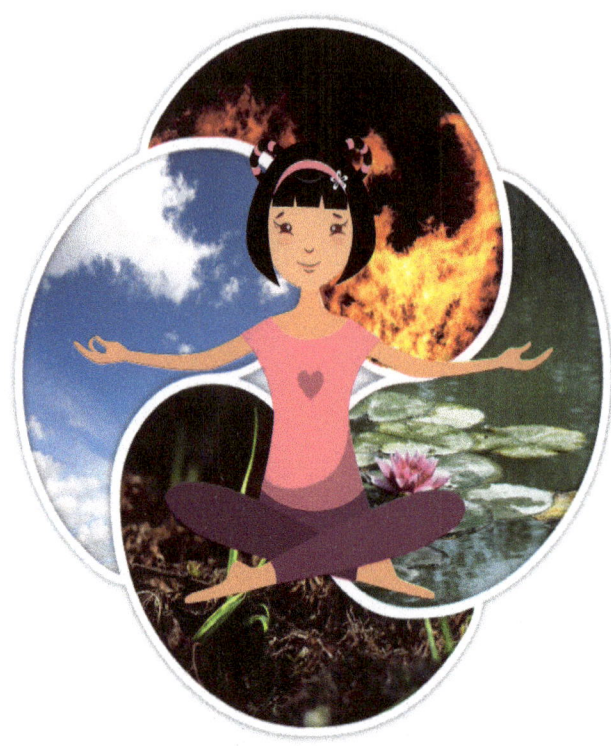

"Connecting with the earth, water, fire, and air elements within us helps to connect with all of nature that surrounds us."

The human body is composed of the *Four Elements,* in varying proportions. The following is where each of the Four Elements are primarily found in the human body:

1. Earth

- Muscles, tissues, bones, joints, teeth, hair, nails, connective tissue, and cells.

2. Water

- Fluids inside the body: blood, plasma, lymph, mucus, urine, sweat, tears, and all the water contained in our cells.

3. Fire

- The digestive system (digestive fire) - digestive enzymes and secretions, and all enzymes.
- Metabolism and the energy in the body brought by our food and used by our body.

4. Air

- The air we breathe (body's breath) and all the gasses that are part of biological and chemical processes of the body.

Crystals that Deepen the Connection with the Four Elements

The Kind Karma Kids Yoga Inner Shaman Practice teaches us how to work with the energy of crystals for: personal use, during yoga practice, class lesson planning & deepening the connection with Mother Earth

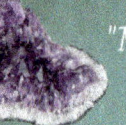

"Make a conscious effort to open your heart & mind to the power of crystal healing"

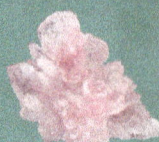

ELEMENT	CRYSTALS ASSOCIATED WITH THE ELEMENT
Earth Element Crystals — Use for growth, grounding & stabilizing energies	Amber, Black Agate, Black Obsidian, Black Onyx, Black Tourmaline, Emerald, Halite (Rock Salt), Hematite, Iron Pyrite, Jade, Jasper, Lava Stone, Malachite, Moss Agate, Petrified Wood, Smoky Quartz, Tree Agate, Tiger's Eye
Water Element Crystals — Use for increasing self-love, kindness & friendships	Amazonite, Aqua Aura Quartz, Aquamarine, Blue Calcite, Blue Lace Agate, Chrysoprase, Epidote, Green Aventurine, Kunzite, Larimar, Lemurian Aquatine Calcite, Lepidolite, Moonstone, Morganite, Opal, Pink Tourmaline, Rose Quartz, Turquoise, Watermelon Tourmaline
Fire Element Crystals — Use for increasing alertness, energy & creativity	Agate, Carnelian, Citrine, Fire Agate, Fire Opal, Golden Labradorite, Honey Calcite, Pyrite, Red Garnet, Red Jasper, Ruby, Sunstone, Tangerine Quartz, Tiger's Eye, Yellow Jasper, Yellow & Orange Tourmaline
Air Element Crystals — Use for mental clarity, reducing brain fog & meditation	Amethyst, Angel Aura Quartz, Angelite, Blue Apatite, Blue Calcite, Blue Kyanite, Blue Quartz, Celestite, Clear Quartz, Danburite, Dumortierite, Fluorite, Iolite, Lepidolite, Rainbow Fluorite, Shungite, Sodalite, Tanzanite

CREATED BY DEAN TELANO

The Seven Sacred Directions of the Medicine Wheel or Sacred Hoop

The Following are Shamanic approaches for honoring the seven sacred directions within the framework of the Medicine Wheel:

1. Calling in the specific directions.
2. Calling ourselves to the directions.
3. Honoring specific qualities of a direction.
4. Creating a connection with the animal yoga poses or animals in each direction.

Qualities Associated with the Seven Directions

1. <u>North Direction</u>: Winter. Midnight. Cold temperatures. Intuition, understanding. Moon. Air element. White. Elder. Spiritual Body.
2. <u>East Direction</u>: Spring. Sunrise. New beginnings, growth. Seedling plants. Sun. Fire element. Yellow. Childhood. Mental body.
3. <u>South Direction</u>: Summer. Midday. Abundance, vitality, maturity. Mother Earth. Water Element. Red. Adolescence. Physical body.
4. <u>West Direction</u>: Autumn. Sunset. Letting go, trust, faith. Earth Element. Black. Adulthood. Emotional body.
5. <u>As Above</u>: Cosmic flow, galaxies, stars. Future, possibility, expanded consciousness. Angels. Ascended masters. God.
6. <u>So Below</u>: Planetary flows & cycles. Collective history, past, fertility, creation. Ancestors & ancestral energies. Goddess.
7. <u>As Within</u>: Now moment, sacredness of being present. Timeless. Openness. We are the connection to above & below. All colors, rainbows. Integration of all bodies.

CREATED BY DEAN TELANO

Key Aspects of the Medicine Wheel for Lesson Plans

DIRECTION	North	East	South	West
SEASON	Winter	Spring	Summer	Autumn
ELEMENT	Air	Fire	Water	Earth
COLOR	White	Yellow	Red	Black
STAGE OF LIFE	Elder	Childhood	Adolescence	Adulthood
FOUR BODIES	Spiritual Body	Mind Body	Physical Body	Emotional Body

This Table is Useful for Creating Class Themes or Lesson Plans. For Yoga Animal Poses: Refer to the Medicine Wheel Illustrations for the Animals in Each of the Four Directions.

References

Yoga
- Telano, Dean. / Kind Karma Yoga. (2020). *Fundamentals of Kind Karma® Yoga. (3rd ed.).*
    Kind Karma Publications

- Telano, Dean. / Kind Karma Yoga. (2022). *Kind Karma Kids Yoga Manual.*
    Kind Karma Publications

Meditation
- Telano, Dean. / Awaken with Meditation. (2020-2021). *Mind-Of-Clear-Light Meditation Manual Vol. I, II, III: Calming the Mind; Calming the Heart; Calming the Spirit. (2nd ed.).*

- Telano, Dean. / Awaken with Meditation. (2022). *Awaken with Meditation Manual: Open Your Heart to Calm Your Mind.*

Crystal Healing
- Telano, Dean. / Kind Karma Inc. (2021). *Kind Karma Crystal Healing Manual. (2nd ed.).*

- Telano, Dean. / Kind Karma Inc. (2022). *Learn Kind Karma Crystal Magic Booklet.*

Blogs
- Telano, Dean. (2021, December, 13). "Kind Karma Worldwide". *Infinity Breathing. Kind Karma® Kids Breathing Exercise for Improving Academic Skills & Focus.* https://www.kindkarmaworldwide.org/post/infinity-breathing-kind-karma-kids-breathing-exercise-for-improving-academic-skills-focus

- Telano, Dean. (2021, December, 23). "Kind Karma Worldwide". *Kind Karma® Crystals for Kindness: Celestite. Raise your Vibes!* https://www.kindkarmaworldwide.org/post/kind-karma-crystals-for-kindness-celestite-raise-your-vibes

About the Author

Dean Telano, Ph.D., E-RYT 500, RCYT, RPYT, YACEP

Author of *"Kind Karma Worldwide™: Inspirational Quotes & Empowering Thoughts for Raising the Vibration of Humanity"*

Founder of *Kind Karma Worldwide™, nonprofit organization*

Creator of *Kind Karma® Yoga, Awaken with Meditation, Awaken Qigong, Kind Karma® Kids Yoga*

Dean is at the forefront of leading others to heal through yoga, sound, crystal therapy, movement meditation, qigong and reiki healing. He holds two master degrees; one in Exercise Physiology, and the other in Yoga Education with a focus on Prenatal Yoga and Children's Yoga. His MS degree in Exercise Physiology paved the path of extensive involvement in the health and fitness fields, nutrition, yoga, meditation, sound healing, and energy work for the past 40 years. Additionally, he is a former adjunct professor, author, exercise physiologist, Medical Qigong Therapist, and Gong Master.

Dean has been certifying students in yoga and meditation since 2001. Graduates from Kind Karma® Yoga are currently teaching all over the world. Kind Karma® Yoga is a heart based and midline integrated yoga that includes powerful core techniques and Rahini Yoga® Kriyas that promote healing and personal empowerment.

As a co-owner of *Kind Karma Yoga & Holistic Center,* Dean shares his wealth of knowledge by teaching and leading courses, seminars, events, and classes that emphasize wellness as a holistic integration of the physical, mental, and spiritual well-being. The programs offered to the public include Yoga, Meditation, Gong and Sound Therapy,

Awaken Qigong, Crystal Healing, and Reiki Healing courses including Crystal Reiki and Animal & Pet Reiki. As a Certified Crystal Healing Practitioner, Ethereal Crystal Reiki Master, and Nature Shaman Reiki Master, Dean offers classes and trainings to the public on crystal healing and tapping into the power traits of animals, nature and the elemental realms for guidance and direction for one's life path.

Registered Yoga Teacher with Yoga Alliance since 2001, Dean's yoga training and study include Kind Karma®Yoga, Rahini Yoga®, Hatha, Kundalini, Vinyasa, Power, Raja, Kundalini Maha, Tibetan, Naam, Yin, MEM Gong Yoga, Restorative and Therapeutic Yoga, and Prenatal and Children's Yoga. His training & experience in meditation includes Shamatha, Zhine, Mantra, Mindfulness, Dzogchen, Zen, Awaken Qigong and Mindful Movement Meditation.

Dean Telano's Kind Karma® Kids Yoga Program has become an inspiring and useful resource for many children of all ages, teachers and all others using yoga as a path to assist the emotional, mental and physical development of children. Kind Karma® Kids Yoga Teacher Trainings are offered through his wellness center, virtually, and to schools to certify and train their teachers and faculty members.

The Kind Karma® Kids Yoga curriculum consists of unique techniques to help children gain strength, positivity, self-esteem, mindfulness, better coping skills and more, through yoga poses, pranayama, meditation and mindfulness, and gong and sound therapy for all ages. Specific and unique to Kind Karma® Kids Yoga, crystals, animals and nature connectivity are incorporated with yoga poses to foster a stronger connection to the pose, the animal prana power, and healing from crystals.

Dean visits colleges and universities teaching Mindfulness Meditation to students and their faculty; as well, travels offering lectures, events and workshops in support of his humanitarian nonprofit organization, **Kind Karma Worldwide**™, *with its mission to raise the consciousness of humanity and the world's vibration.*

To learn more about Dr. Dean Telano, visit his website:

https://www.deantelano.com

CONTACTS

For more information on Dr. Dean Telano, Kind Karma® Yoga & Kind Karma Worldwide™ - *Humanitarian Nonprofit 501(c)(3) Organization*, **visit:**

- **DR. DEAN TELANO**
  www.deantelano.com
  Learn how to achieve vibrant health, nourish your mind, body and soul and live a high vibrational life through the many programs and certifications Dr. Dean Telano offers.

- **KIND KARMA® YOGA**
  www.kindkarmayoga.com
  Learn about Kind Karma Yoga, Kind Karma Kids Yoga, Kind Karma Yin Yoga, and Awaken with Meditation.

- **KIND KARMA WORLDWIDE™**
  www.kindkarmaworldwide.org
  Learn more about Dr. Dean Telano's Humanitarian Nonprofit 501(c)(3) Organization and its 4 Initiatives.

- **KIND KARMA YOGA & HOLISTIC CENTER**
  www.kindkarmaholistic.com
  Dr. Dean Telano is a co-owner of Kind Karma Yoga & Holistic Center. This wellness center provides yoga & meditation classes for all ages, including virtual options, holistic training programs and services.

Available for PURCHASE on Amazon

"Kind Karma Worldwide™: *Inspirational Quotes & Empowering Thoughts for Raising the Vibration of Humanity*": authored by Dr. Dean Telano

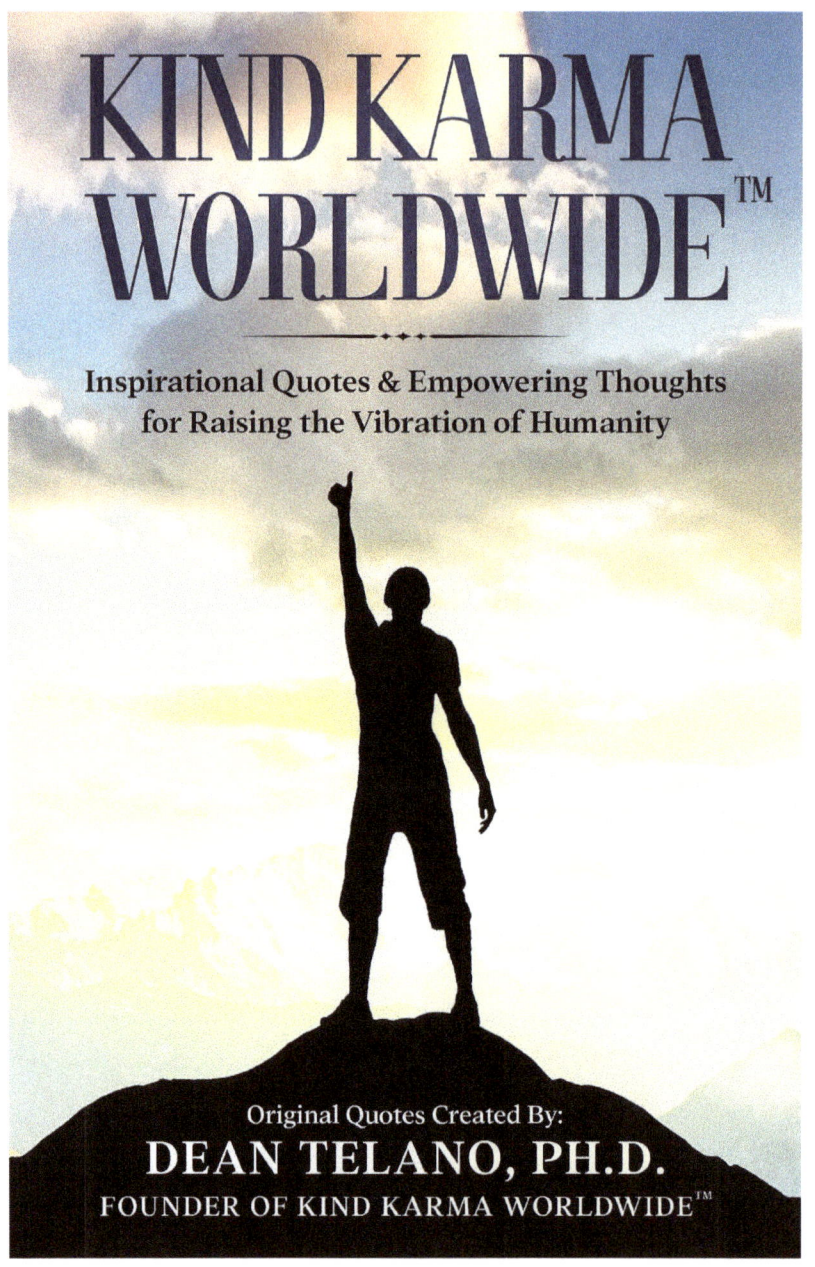

PURCHASE
Kind Karma Cares Bears

To support the *Kind Karma Cares Initiative* that provides noninvasive energy therapies for sick, abused, sheltered, farm and domesticated animals.

Your support will have a lasting impact on the world today!

Kind Karma Worldwide™
Humanitarian Nonprofit Organization

Support Kind Karma Worldwide™
Purchase a Kind Karma® Cares Bears

All Kind Karma® Cares Bears are Infused with Kind Karma Reiki, Angelic & Shamanic Healing Energy

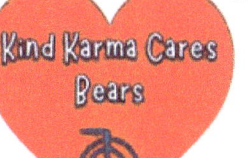
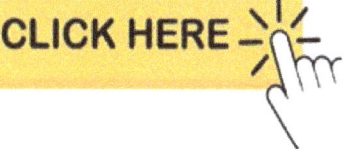

To order your Kind Karma Reiki Cares Bears, visit
www.kindkarmaworldwide.org

www.ingramcontent.com/pod-product-compliance
Lightning Source LLC
Chambersburg PA
CBHW061811290426
44110CB00026B/2850